=04

D0486538

THE LIMITS AND LIES OF
HUMAN GENETIC RESEARCH

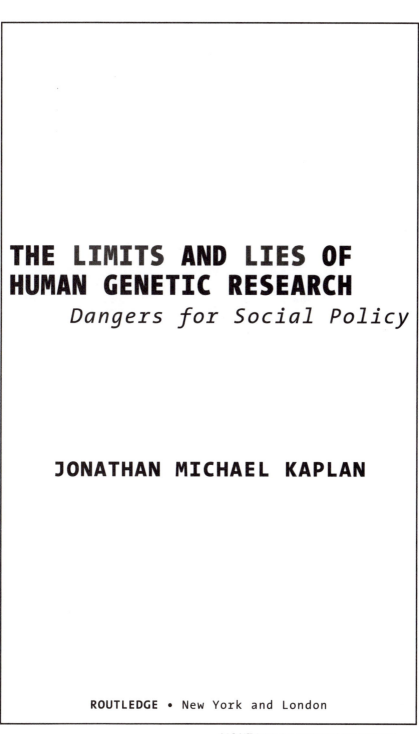

THE LIMITS AND LIES OF HUMAN GENETIC RESEARCH
Dangers for Social Policy

JONATHAN MICHAEL KAPLAN

ROUTLEDGE • New York and London

MONTROSE LIBRARY DISTRICT
320 So. 2nd St.
Montrose, CO 81401

Published in 2000 by
Routledge
29 West 35th Street
New York, NY 10001

Published in Great Britain by
Routledge
11 New Fetter Lane
London EC4P 4EE

Copyright © 2000 by Routledge

Printed in the United States of America on acid-free paper.

All rights reserved. No part of this book may be reprinted or reproduced or utilized in any form or by any electronic, mechanical or other means, now known or here-after invented, including photocopying and recording or in any information storage or retrieval system, without permission in writing from the publishers.

Library of Congress Cataloging-in-Publication Data
Kaplan, Jonathan Michael.
  The limits and lies of human genetic research : dangers for social policy / by Jonathan Michael Kaplan.
    p. cm. —(Reflective bioethics)
Includes bibliographical references and index.
ISBN 0-415-92637-8 (hb. : acid-free paper) — ISBN 0-415-92638-6 (pb. : acid-free paper)
  1. Medical genetics—Moral and ethical aspects. 2. Human genetics—Research—Moral and ethical aspects. 3. Human genetics—Research—social aspects. I. Title. II. Series.
RB155 .K36 2000
17f4'.28—dc21   99-044899

Designed by Cynthia Dunne

CONTENTS

LIST OF FIGURES AND BOXES

Figures

Boxes

ACKNOWLEDGMENTS

I f there has been any one idea guiding my work in philosophy over the past decade, it is that we are *social* beings. No work, however small, is ever the product of any single individual. In working on this book, it was my joy and privilege to be surrounded by family, friends, and colleagues, without whom this project would obviously have been impossible.

I'd first like to thank John Dupré, whose confidence in the original project and encouragement were unwavering, and without whom this work would never have been begun, let alone finished. Not only does his work provide much of the background and inspiration for this project, but it stands as an example of just how important, and relevant, philosophy of science with a political bent can be.

Debra Satz has also been involved with this project since its conception, and without her this project would have been at best a pale shadow of what it is now. My thanks; whatever and however deep our philosophical disagreements, I have always found our areas of agreement to be much more important.

My friend Eric Schulman deserves a special note of thanks as well. He too has been involved in this project since the beginning, albeit as an outsider to philosophy. Nevertheless, his help has ranged from the early conceptualizations of the work as a whole to careful readings of several drafts of the entire manuscript, and again, without his input, the work would have been very different, and much worse. More than that, though, my friendship with Eric has been one of the most important in my life, and I cannot imagine the person I would be were it not for him.

Alan Nelson not only read and commented helpfully on various drafts of this work, but has been a valued friend, mentor, and collaborator throughout my philosophical career. Without his encouragement, and, more importantly, his example, I very much doubt that I would still be doing philosophy today.

Jim Nelson also read and commented on various drafts of this work. His comments have always been helpful and positive, and I thank him for them.

Peter Godfrey-Smith's trenchant criticisms of early versions of this work helped keep me honest throughout, and he made many useful suggestions as well. If not for his criticisms, as well as his help developing many of the examples used in chapters 3 and 4, the work would undoubtedly be less rigorous and more open to charges of sloppiness. Any mistakes or confusions that still exist in those chapters are, of course, my own, but without Peter there would surely have been many more of them.

While Michael Blake, Timothy Crocket, Avrom Faderman, Lisa Mcleod, and Matthew Price all read and commented on drafts. I'd mostly like to thank them for their friendship and support over our time together. Stephan Käufer not only read and commented on early drafts of several chapters, but has also been a valued collaborator in other contexts as well as a valued friend.

Steffan Sonck and Janet Stemwedel helped me work through some of the technical aspects of this material, and I'd like to thank them both for their time, as well as their patience with my inability to grasp what must have seemed to them to be very simple concepts. Janet also read and commented usefully on substantial portions of the manuscript.

Ina Roy read and commented helpfully on early drafts of several chapters. Elizabeth Anderson made several helpful suggestions at the beginning of this project. My conversations with Tim Schroeder were a valuable source of inspiration, and he found several excellent examples I've used in the book. Steve Downes and David Magnus read the entire manuscript and made many helpful suggestions. Doug Maclean's comments were very helpful and insightful, and an anonymous reader made significant contributions as well.

There are various philosophers whose work I relied upon more than most in thinking through the issues I confront here. As will be obvious to anyone who reads this book, R. C. Lewontin's work was central to my thinking on many, if not most, of these issues, and I owe him an enormous debt for doing the work that made this work possible. I am only half joking when I say that if more people had read and understood his seminal work on these issues (much of it done in the 1970s) this book would be unnecessary. It will also be clear to the reader that I have relied very heavily on the recent work of Massimo Pigliucci and Carl Schlichting.

Massimo I would also like to thank for many interesting discussions of these issues and for his comments and criticisms, especially on chapters 2, 3, and 4. Again, any confusions that remain in those chapters are my own, but without Massimo's help there would have been many more. While not so quite so obvious, my exposure to the work of Feyerabend and Wittgenstein informed my work on this project from the start, and without that influence I would not be the sort of philosopher I am.

Finally, I'd like to thank my parents, Loretta Francesco and Martin Kaplan. Their vast and unwavering support was more often than not all that prevented my utter failure; any small success I've achieved in life I owe entirely to them. I cannot express my love and gratitude deeply enough.

No list such as this is ever complete. Many other people have been a help in this project, either by reading early drafts, or by being around when I needed them, and often by both. If there is anything of value in this work at all it is only because so many people supported me throughout the process; too many, alas, to name.

Where to end such a list is always at some level an arbitrary decision, and it always involves not acknowledging some debt. But acknowledged or not, those people to whom I owe these debts of gratitude know they can collect whenever, and however often, they wish.

CHAPTER 1

EXPLAINING DIFFERENCES

Differences That Make a Difference

This book is primarily about the differences between people, and the stories that we tell to explain these differences. That people are different, and different in ways that matter to us, is obvious. But the reasons that people differ from each other are not so obvious, and explanations for these differences vary by culture, by time, and by the individual or group offering the explanation. In the United States, explanations that revolve around genetics and make appeals to our genes have been popular for some time. While explanations appealing to genes have suffered the occasional setback, their popularity has been on the rise in recent years. Over the past decade, there has been an increase both in the number and in the boldness of explanations that attribute the differences between people (both physical and behavioral) to the genetic variations between them.

Explanations of human variation do not occur in a vacuum; the cause of variation in complex traits is explored because people think it is worthwhile, and the explanations that are generated are put to various uses. Sometimes they are used quite literally in social and political discussions; at other times, the way these considerations are brought to bear on various issues is more subtle. But in either case, the force of such explanations extends beyond their obvious domains and into the domains of various political and social issues. In these different domains, explanations premised on the importance of genetic differences have changed not only the sorts of considerations that are brought to bear on the political and social issues, but have also helped to determine the kinds of outcomes considered reasonable.

How do these kinds of explanations, explanations of differences that primarily refer to genetic differences, change the sorts of considerations brought to bear, and the outcomes considered reasonable, in the discussions and debates that surround political and social issues? In this work, I argue that explanations of this sort do at least the following things: they increase our tendency to view the traits involved in these explanations as real (a reification of the traits in question); they make the explanations appear to arise not out of contingent and contestable social organizations but out of the natural order of things (a naturalization of the traits in question); and they create and reinforce expectations about the proper perspective from which to view such issues as modifications to the traits in question. These changes constitute a change in the discourse that surrounds these traits, and the issues wrapped up in them. But why are such explanations popular? How are these explanations supposed to work? Does the research purporting to support such explanations really do so? What other kinds of explanations could account for these differences, given the available evidence about their causes?

There are any number of ways one could go about answering these and similar questions. Here I approach answering these questions in two ways. First, I look at genetic explanations of differences in both behaviors and physical attributes generally, in order to understand the strengths and the weaknesses of the techniques used in contemporary human genetic research. Then I explore the research that has been done in six different areas that seem to be important to us, at least as a culture if not necessarily as individuals. That these areas involve issues that are generally seen as important is revealed in part by the amount of media attention the traits wrapped up in the issues generate, as well as the attention paid to them by researchers interested in explaining their causes. In some of the cases, such as explanations for differences in rates of violent crime or the causal history of medical conditions like clinical depression, the reasons for the high levels of interest are relatively easy to understand. In other cases, such as sexual orientation, it is harder to see why the traits in question have generated the level of interest that they have. Part of understanding why genetic explanations are popular in these cases will involve trying to get clear on why these traits are of interest at all, and what role attempting to "explain" them has within our culture.

In the end, I argue against accepting the role that genetic explanations often play in these cases. The reasons I argue why we should reject these explanations differ in the different cases, though. There is no *one* reason why we should reject these explanations, and no argument is given to a general conclusion that all such explanations *must* be wrong. Rather, I argue that we ought to consider each case on its own merits, and strive to understand the similarities and the differences that each individual case might have to other issues we've confronted before. In some cases, it will turn out that we should reject the explanations given in terms of genetics because the research cited as supporting the explanations simply doesn't do so. In other cases, even if the research is technically impeccable, it emerges out of a perspective that is itself questionable; change the assumptions, and the very point of the research can vanish, leaving barren technical results with no social or policy implications at all.

But rejecting explanations in terms of genetic differences in these cases shouldn't lead to immediately accepting other explanations either. Attempting to explain those differences in terms of environmental differences would also be a mistake. In the cases that follow, it will turn out that claims of that sort are unsupportable as well. Some people may be unhappy being told that we currently have *no* explanation that is adequate in these cases; however, I think it is unarguable that, at least as far as policy decisions are concerned, we do more harm, and make more tragic mistakes, when we accept bad explanations than when we admit that we simply don't know what the right answer is. In large part, this work will be arguing that for many of the questions that matter to us at the intersection of human differences and social policy, we simply don't know what the right answer is, nor even how to go about figuring it out.

The Ascension of the Genetic

Gene Discovery May Yield Test for Glaucoma . . .
Brain-Tied Gene Defect May Explain Why
    Schizophrenics Hear Voices . . .
Finding Genetic Traces of Jewish Priesthood . . .
People Haunted by Anxiety Appear to Be Short on a Gene . . .
Scientists Identify Site of Gene Tied to Some Cases of Parkinson's . . .
Gene May Be Clue to Nature of Nurturing . . .
Researchers Track Down a Gene That
    May Govern Spatial Abilities . . .
Variant Gene Tied to Love of New Thrills . . .

It is hard to open a newspaper and not see headlines like the above.[1] With each week, if not each day, there seems to be a new announcement. A gene is found for a trait, either physical or behavioral (though rarely is a well-understood pathway from the gene to the trait known), an association is found between some genetic variation and some trait (although the gene itself has not been located or sequenced), variation in a trait is found to have some genetic component (though no gene has been found), or a story about how genes must be at the heart of something is told (though no gene has been found and no genetic component to variation demonstrated).

Walter Gilbert thinks that three different questions are raised by the current possibilities in genetics research (1992, 84). At the most general level, there is a question about how human beings (or for that matter any sophisticated multicellular organism) develop from a fertilized egg into their adult form (a question about developmental biology generally). A more specific question asks how that developmental process differs between different complex organisms (between, for example, humans and other primates). Finally, at the most specific level, we might wonder "how do we differ from one another?" (84). Plomin et al. make a similar point when they claim that the most specific questions, questions about differences *within* a species, are those that "most often confront scientists studying human behavior" and those which "genetics . . . is uniquely qualified to aid us in analyzing" (1990, 9–11).

Plomin et al. go on to point out that "the behavioral issues of greatest relevance to society are issues of individual differences" (246) and that it is "the study of things that make a difference: the description, prediction, explanation, and alteration of individual differences" that drive "societal interest in the behavioral sciences" (247). While there is certainly some intellectual interest in such things as the answers to Gilbert's first two questions, it is really the promise of answers to questions of the third sort that generates "societal interest" (and with such interest, funding). But it is, of course, only some of the individual differences that "make a difference." Researchers have not been inspired to spend time and money trying to account for many of the traits that vary between people, such as, for example, our particular tastes in food and clothing. And some projects that have been undertaken (e.g., measuring the heritability of height: see Plomin et al. 1990, 320) have aroused relatively little interest or controversy. The issues at the heart of things are, indeed, those that involve the promise to explain, predict, and control what are generally thought of as, in one way or another, important, and often behavioral, differences.[2] It is the hope of being able to predict and control such things as intelligence, mental illness, alcoholism (and other "addictive behaviors'), "criminal" behavior, violent behaviors, obesity, and the like, that make the promise of human genetic research so tempting.

Relatively recent advances made in genetic research have been instrumental in contemporary work in gene mapping (finding where on the human genome—on what chromosome and where on that chromo-some—a gene correlated with a trait is located) and gene sequencing (finding the sequence of base-pairs in the gene[s] in question). The cre-ation of these sets of modern abilities has created a flurry of interest in mapping and sequencing genes correlated with various traits, so far mostly genetic diseases. However, results have begun to emerge in research into the genetic bases of some behavioral traits, and other com-plex traits, including those considered part of normal human variation.

Much of the current excitement in the search for genetic explanations for variation in complex human traits comes out of the possibility of using those techniques that have emerged from the concentration of resources into molecular genetics to study the traits in question. The hope is that the sort of gene finding and gene sequencing that is becoming increas-ingly feasible with respect to physical diseases will make equally plausible the explication of the genetic bases of those variations in, for example, behaviors in human populations that have a partial genetic etiology. However, as we shall see, finding, sequencing, and tracing the pathways from the purported genes to the behavioral traits of interest has proven difficult for researchers in human behavior genetics, who for the most part have therefore had to content themselves with studies that attempt to show merely that there is a genetic component to human behavioral vari-ation in some instance, and to give some estimate of the extent of the genetic influence on that variation. And, I will argue, even when researchers do find genes associated with variations in complex traits, it is often difficult to know what to make of this. Using this information to make predictions or give certain kinds of explanations is very difficult at best, and often impossible.

The techniques for estimating the extent of the role of genetic differ-ences in the variation in various traits have serious limitations, however. When used in ordinary human populations, the maximum accuracy that can be expected from these methods is fairly low. And the techniques have serious conceptual limitations, which put fundamental limits on the proper interpretations of any results achieved. Attempting to make use of these results without fully acknowledging their limitations will be revealed as a major source of errors, errors that lead to very dubious argu-ments about the role of genetic differences in framing discussions about issues of public policy and social justice.

Here is where I hope the force of this work will be felt. The rise of the popularity of these kinds of genetic explanations wouldn't be very impor-tant if these explanations weren't linked to political and social issues that matter. Whether the explanations followed from good research or bad, whether the interpretations of the research were legitimate or not, whether the research itself relied on culturally contingent assumptions that could be undermined or not—none of these questions would be of interest outside a narrow set of scientists and people interested in the study of science if it weren't for the links between these kinds of explanations and social policy choices. But once we see what the limits of these implications really are, what the research can and cannot show, and how easy misinterpretations are to make (as well as how they can be avoided), the claimed policy implications will look much more questionable, and in many cases will be revealed to be best discounted entirely. With the limits of these kinds of genetic explanations displayed, the room will be created for other considerations—many of which speak in directions different from the genetic—to influence our views of these issues.

The Six Arenas

The goal of this work, then, is to demonstrate that the rise of explanations premised on the importance of the genetic to explain many the differences in behaviors and physical characteristics that we find important has inappropriately influenced our views of issues that matter to us. Conversely, certain views of these issues—that is, certain kinds of purported solutions—make the appropriation of genetic research to do political work both more likely and rather more dangerous than do other views. The work of demonstrating these points is done primarily through a series of case studies, each of which shows in a different way how human genetic research has influenced, and how the interpretation of such research has been influenced by, specific kinds of political and social issues in contemporary society.

The first cases examined are narrowly focused on the use of human genetic research in supporting claims about social policies. In chapter 4 I discuss some of the history behind arguments surrounding race, socioeconomic status, and average IQ scores. Arguments from the supposed high heritability of intelligence and the disparities in average IQ scores between various "races" to the conclusion that it is genetic differences that drive these disparities, have a long and ignoble history. In analyzing both the traditional and more modern counterarguments, I attempt to make clear what sorts of errors most often get made in this form of research and how these mistakes interact with the technical limitations of the research used. More recent research attempting to find genes associated with scores on IQ tests is also critiqued. Both the broadest conclusions that I argue for in that chapter—namely, that neither heritability estimates in human populations for complex traits nor molecular-level associations between genes and such traits are in the least bit useful for making policy decisions unless huge numbers of unargued-for (and for the most part insupportable) assumptions are made—and the more detailed analyses of how technical results in human behavior genetics are often misunderstood and misused, will inform the rest of the work.

Next I explore the way in which genetic research into the causes of criminality and violence has been instrumental in defining individuals and delineating the bounds of discourse around the issues. Specifically, in focusing on causation at the level of individual differences, such research detracts attention from wider environmental differences. The next chapter, on research into the genetics of sexual orientation, more directly confronts the issue of the interaction of the social construction of behavioral traits and ways of organizing behaviors within a culture with research into possible genetic bases for those traits.

The next chapters move to a more general level of analysis. In the case of the medicalization of mood-affective disorders, the focus of the chapter is on the use of genetic models to create the clinically depressed as a type of individual and to locate the illness within the individual. This, I argue, makes certain forms of social critique difficult or impossible. A similar argument is made in the next chapter, on obesity, although in this case there is an additional wrinkle, namely that the research that purports to show obesity as a dangerous disease is itself problematic, irrespective of the research into the causes of obesity.

Finally, I turn to a yet higher level of analysis. I argue that the current debates and discussions surrounding contract pregnancies, so-called surrogate mother contracts, as well as the law that is emerging from the legal cases involving such contracts, point toward the creation of the genetic as primary to parenthood in a way both insupportable by genetic research narrowly construed and destructive to many important social considerations about what it means to be a parent. The movement in law toward treating genetic parenthood as the most important criterion when making decisions about the legal rights and obligations associated with parenthood could not, I argue, be made without the overblown rhetoric of contemporary genetic research, and the effects of this movement can only be destructive to other, perhaps more useful, ways of conceiving of parenthood within this culture. This section deals with the genetic influence in much broader and more general terms than the others, since there is no one research program being alluded to when there is a legal ruling that, for example, someone who is the genetic but not gestational mother should get the legal rights and obligations associated with parenthood, and the gestational but not genetic mother should be denied those rights and obligations. This kind of influence, diffuse though it sometimes seems, is important to understanding how the more narrow research projects discussed previously get a rhetorical power and force that extends well beyond their immediate results.

A Few General Observations

For a combination of historical reasons growing out of the development of modern evolutionary theory, conceptual reasons having to do with the technical limitations of certain techniques used in genetic research, and more broadly cultural reasons having to do with contemporary views of the social and political landscape, the environment (especially the social environment) often tends to be viewed as rather more stable and unchanging than a dispassionate view would take it to be, at least within the contexts of these sorts of research projects. And this is important, because a view that takes the social and political landscape to be stable supports the status quo in a particularly devious manner.

The sorts of research projects that are undertaken and the way that these projects are interpreted and appropriated for political ends are influenced by the ways that we think about our relationship to our environment—both our cultural environment and our environment more generally. In displaying this tendency for specific cases, and in providing some general tools for understanding why this is so often the case and what kinds of effects it is likely to have, I hope this book points not toward an automatic rejection of one form of explanation and acceptance of another, but instead toward a way of thinking carefully about the relationship different kinds of explanations have to our ways of thinking about policy. Sometimes we may think that explanations given about the causes of variation are relevant and important to social policy considerations; at other times, however, we may well realize that the explanations are misleading in important ways and ought to be ignored when it comes to making public policy decisions.

It is this kind of complexity and sophistication, I believe, that we need to make sense of this world and problems we face within it.

CHAPTER 2
VARIETIES OF DETERMINISM

Determinism and Determinisms

Almost without exception, those people who write or speak about the relationship between genetics and human traits want to deny that they support "genetic determinism." However, this denial is often made against a background of deep confidence in the importance of genetic research for understanding and controlling those traits that matter to us. This confidence sometimes results in researchers saying and writing things that, at least on the face of it, certainly seem to support various theses that have a deterministic ring to them. Much of this book is concerned with very specific claims, such as those about the relationship between particular research projects and social issues. But those specific claims emerge out of a background of faith in the relative importance of genetics and the relative lack of importance of the environment in explaining variations in traits that matter to us. Revealing this background, I hope, will help make clear the assumptions that lie behind the claims made by those researchers discussed in later chapters.

In what follows, then, I will try to bring out what researchers understand themselves to be denying when they deny that they support or believe in genetic determinism, and the tensions between these denials and the researchers' stated beliefs about the importance of genes and genetic research for understanding and controlling human traits. On the one hand, it will turn out that there are some versions of genetic determinism that no one supports (at least when they are being careful); on the other, there are some versions that seem to have wide support. In going through some researchers' vigorous denials that they support genetic determinism, some of these possible forms of genetic determinism will be explored.

Next, the story of the genetic disease PKU (phenylketonuria) will be told as a way of examining how these points play out in practice. Here the tension between many writers' and researchers' firm belief in the centrality of the gene both causally and methodologically and their stand against naive forms of genetic determinism will be explored. PKU has become the main example used to deny genetic determinism and delineate the limits of the power of genes with respect to phenotypic variations. The history of this disease, however, has traditionally been rewritten as a story about the power and centrality of the genetic for understanding, predicting, and modifying human phenotypic variations (including behavior). In other words, I will argue that a story that was supposed to show that genetic determinism is false is in fact usually written to make PKU seem far more deterministically genetic and the genetic far more important to explaining, predicting, and controlling the disease than a more careful reading of the history of the disease would permit. Seeing how and why this rewriting occurred is a fascinating entry into how the tension plays out in practice between the conviction that genes are at the "heart" of things (as, for example, Watson would have it; see Watson 1992, 167) and the conviction that genetic determinism must be denied.

Against Genetic Determinism?

What exactly the thesis of genetic determinism is meant to claim is rarely made explicit, especially in the writings of the various researchers and popular writers who state their unequivocal opposition to it. But in denying the thesis of genetic determinism various researchers and other writers make various sorts of claims, and from these claims some ideas about the form of the thesis they are arguing against can be gleaned. The claims these researchers make when standing against genetic determinism, however, sometimes rest uneasily with the claims they put forward when discussing the results and likely benefits of the research they undertake. This section stresses the general tension that results when one attempts to deny a form of genetic determinism while simultaneously engaging in research that is premised on the centrality of genes, and perhaps the deterministic, but at the very least predictable, nature of the pathways between genes and physical or behavioral traits (the pathways between genotype and phenotype).

How, then, do researchers stand against genetic determinism, and what is it they stand against when they do so? One strand of genetic determinism that researchers oppose could be described as the "complete information" strand. Genetic determinism, on this reading of the thesis, would claim that everything about us (including, on some interpretations, our behavior) is predictable, or at least in some way determined or dictated by our genes. So Gilbert, in his much-quoted "A Vision of the Grail," states that "genetic information does *not* dictate everything about us" and that this sort of "shallow genetic determinism is unwise and untrue" (1992, 96). Plomin et al. state that "genes do not determine one's destiny" and that they are not "master puppeteers . . . pulling our strings" (1990, 9). Kagan, in his book detailing his research into the heritability of temperament, notes that the "power of genes is real but limited" and "development is a cooperative mission and no behavior is a first-order, direct product of genes" (1994, 37). This strand of genetic determinism, however, is generally (and quite properly) regarded as trivially false, and very little work is done arguing against it.

A more common reading of the thesis of genetic determinism, and one that makes it at least a bit less outrageous, is that for traits with a genetic etiology, environmental interventions are useless: if a trait is genetic, one is (going to be) stuck with it. This might be called the "intervention is useless" strand.[1] So Dawkins, of *Selfish Gene* fame, stands against genetic determinism in a letter published in *Nature* by objecting to "the suggestion that we are stuck with our biological nature and can't change it" (Dawkins 1981, 528). Wilson, a founder of "sociobiology," also in a letter in *Nature*, writes of the possible genetic basis of xenophobia that "a knowledge of such a hereditary basis can lead to the circumvention of destructive behavior such as racism" (Wilson 1981, 627). Hamer and Copeland note that while "many core personality traits are inherited at birth," this doesn't mean that "people are "stuck" with their personalities from birth" (Hamer and Copeland 1998, 6, 7). Bouchard, of Minnesota Twin Study fame, notes in one of his many articles in *Science* that "intervention is not precluded even for highly heritable traits" (Bouchard et al. 1994, 228), about as pro forma a stand against this strand of genetic determinism as one can take, but still a stand against it. Breakefield, a researcher doing work on the genetic basis of violence, says that people with the "right type of support" often do just fine, even when they have a "syndrome" with "major metabolic consequences." "The purpose," she says, "of this kind of research is to discover what that support is, and who needs it" (quoted in Mann 1994, 1689; re research into genetic bases of violence, see also chapter 5). Plomin et al. note that the fact that "heritability does not constrain environmental interventions" is a "corollary of the point that heritability does not imply genetic determinism" (1997,

85). As we will see in the next section, it is this strand of genetic determinism that the stories surrounding PKU are supposed to put to rest; telling the story of PKU's environmental cure is supposed to display the falsity of genetic determinism by showing that even for traits with genetic etiologies, (environmental) intervention is not useless. For that reason, it is the "intervention is useless" strand of genetic determinism that I will most often be referring to when discussing what it is that researchers who deny genetic determinism take themselves to be denying.

However, we might ask if the "complete information" and "intervention is useless" strands capture all of the forms of genetic determinism that could legitimately go under that name. In what follows, I will try to make it clear that many researchers, even those who are adamantly against being considered genetic determinists, hold that (a) the genetic is the natural place to look when attempting to explain, predict, and control traits with even partial genetic etiologies, and that (b) traits with partial genetic etiologies are best understood as being *primarily* genetic, and it is only through *directed* intervention that the expression of genes for traits with partial genetic etiologies can be avoided or controlled. The first claim is a methodological stance that, at least in principle, can be decoupled from any form of determinism.[2] However, the second claim seems roughly causal in nature, and only likely to be true if, for example, genotype-phenotype pathways are, in "normal" conditions, at least something much like deterministic. For this reason, I think the second is a thesis that should be considered a kind of genetic determinism. While, again, one could hold the methodological thesis without holding the causal thesis, if one holds the causal thesis the methodological thesis will probably be adopted as well. In any event, as we will see in the next section, many people denying genetic determinism seem to hold both the methodological and causal stances discussed above. And indeed, part of the payoff of telling a different kind of story about PKU is seeing that the version of genetic determinism made up of the causal and methodological stances is untenable.

Before moving on, though, it is worth noting that many of the same researchers who attacked genetic determinism in its "intervention is useless" or "complete information" strands make claims about the limits of the genetic that seem to rest uneasily with denials of any form of genetic determinism. Early in Gilbert's "Grail" piece he states that "there is no more basic or more fundamental information that could be available" than our DNA sequence, that it is "the most fundamental property of the body" (1992, 83). Gilbert goes on to claim that our DNA is what "actually specifies the human organism," that it actually answers the question

"What makes us human?" (84). More boldly still, he states that actually being able to hold one's own gene sequence in one's hand (on CD) will "be difficult for humans" since "we look upon ourselves as having an infinite potential" and the recognition "that we are determined . . . by a finite collection of information that is knowable" is the "closing on an intellectual frontier" (96). While nothing here is *strictly* incompatible with denying either the "complete information" or "intervention is useless" strands, there is certainly at least a kind of tension between making these kinds of claims and denying either, let alone both, of those strands. When Watson argues that if one is going to throw money at some large-scale project, large-scale projects related to genetics are a good place to do it, because "genetics lies at the heart of so much" (1992, 167), it is relatively easy to interpret him as not supporting either the "complete information" or the "intervention is useless" strands of genetic determinism (but perhaps only a version of the methodological thesis mentioned above). However, at a conference in 1995 Watson noted that as people get old, their thoughts turn either to "genetics or to God" because they become "interested in their fate" (1995, n.p.), it was rather harder to find an interpretation that didn't at least point in the direction of some version of genetic determinism (either a weak reading of "complete information" involved with prediction, or a reading of "intervention is useless" in that it isn't at all clear how "fates" could be avoided by environmental intervention). And of course, Dawkins's flirtations with genetic determinism are the stuff of legend. No one can forget, from his popular book *The Selfish Gene*, such classics as the claim that we are "robot vehicles blindly programmed to preserve the selfish molecules known as genes" (preface) and that these genes "swarm in huge colonies, safe inside gigantic lumbering robots, sealed off from the outside world . . . manipulating it by remote control." "They are," he finishes, "in you and me; they control us body and mind" (1976, 21). These claims certainly sound as if they give some support to both of the radical strands of genetic determinism discussed above, though perhaps they don't affirm the very strongest available versions of those theses.

PKU: The Traditional Accounts and the History: Determinism through the Back Door

The primary example now used to warn against genetic determinism and to establish the limits of the genetic is that of the genetic disease phenylketonuria (PKU) and its environmental cure. The version of the story that gets told throughout the vast majority of the literature, however, is, both in its broad outline and its details, simplified and misleading, and often simply mistaken. In its standard forms, it has become a central myth of behavioral genetics, told and retold, with its moral (that genetic determinism is false) always taken to be obvious.

It is ironic, then, that the standard story of PKU actually ends up affirming a version of genetic determinism. That which is genetic, in the standard version of the PKU story, is, while perhaps not immutable, modifiable only through massive and directed (and usually medical) intervention (a version of the weaker causal thesis discussed above). Further, the standard story strongly implies that it is by attention to the genetic that one gains the ability to predict, explain, and control many of the behaviors that interest us (a version of the methodological thesis discussed above). The focus of this section is on the way the story of PKU gets twisted from a warning about the limits of the genetic to a tale reaffirming the genetic as central and more than vaguely deterministic.

In what follows, I will bring out the ways in which the variations between the version of the PKU story ordinarily given and a somewhat more detailed and historically accurate account of its discovery, etiology, and treatments are revealing of deep assumptions about the power and centrality of the genetic both within the community of researchers and in their critics. The differences between the "mythical" PKU story and the more historically minded story reveal all too well what a radical version of genetic determinism writers both within and outside of traditional genetic research programs must be standing against when they use the standard version of the PKU story to oppose the thesis. The more historically accurate version supports none of the assumptions about the centrality of the genetic that make their way into the standard account.

The Mythical PKU

It has become traditional to start cautionary tales about the falsity of the thesis of genetic determinism by telling the story of PKU, which is, according to the traditional account, a single-gene defect that is almost entirely correctable through environmental interventions. In the introduction to their text, Plomin et al. provide the standard story of PKU:

> Once in a great while, we find relatively simple genetic and physiological systems. This is what happened for one type of mental retardation, phenylketonuria (PKU), which is caused by a single-gene defect.

A little later they mention,

> [b]iochemical studies of the gene-behavior pathways indicated that the ultimate cause of the retardation was the inability to break down a par-

ticular chemical, phenylalanine, which led to its accumulation at high levels in the blood.

As well, they assert that

> PKU individuals do not suffer retardation if a diet low in phenylalanine is provided during developmental years. Thus, an environmental intervention was successful in bypassing a genetic problem. This important discovery was made possible by recognition of the genetic basis for this particular type of retardation. (Plomin et al. 1990, 8, 9)

For Plomin et al. the story forms an example of the sort of thing research in human behavior genetics will someday let us find all the time— a gene-behavior pathway that we can understand biochemically and then modify with some form of medical intervention.[3] And it is this ability to intervene in the gene-behavior pathway that makes the thesis of genetic determinism false. To be genetic is not to be unmodifiable because, Plomin et al. make clear, a "genetically determined behavioral problem may be bypassed, ameliorated, or remediated by environmental interventions" (1990, 9).[4] And, the story further implies, it is by an attention to, and the understanding of, the genetics involved that we come to be able to understand and control these traits.[5]

It is this message that is conveyed by the stories that get repeated throughout the literature. This version of the PKU myth, in even shorter form, makes an appearance in papers both by authors strongly in favor of increased spending on genetic research and by authors more wary of, for example, the Human Genome Project and its promises. Caskey, in an article explicitly pushing for more research into medicine based on genes and genetic technologies, notes that the ability to "detect severe, treatable inborn errors of metabolism" soon led to "successful prevention of mental retardation from phenylketonuria (PKU)" (1992, 116). Kitcher, in an article for the *New York Times*, noted,

> Children with PKU carry genes that render them unable to metabolize the amino acid phenylalanine. Left untreated, they build up large amounts of phenylalanine in their cells (and lack sufficient amounts of another amino acid, tyrosine) and become severely mentally retarded. By testing a baby just after birth, however, a doctor can prescribe a diet low in phenylalanine and high in tyrosine that enables an afflicted child to develop normally. (1996)

An article by Vigue in *The American Biology Teacher* recounts the classic story in surprising detail (she cites Burns 1993 as the source of her information on PKU):

It is often assumed that traits with the highest heritabilities cannot be modified by the environment. With our burgeoning understanding of how genes work, this assumption is becoming less and less valid. Consider, for example, the mental retardation associated with PKU (phenylketonuria), a disorder caused by a single defective gene. There is no question that PKU is a classic inherited disorder and that the symptoms will develop in almost any normal human environment. Once the mechanisms whereby the PKU gene produces its devastating effects was understood, however, the cure for its symptoms became obvious: PKU is a disorder of phenylalanine metabolism. When phenylalanine is eliminated from the diet of PKU babies, the associated retardation does not develop. . . .

From this, Vigue would have us draw two conclusions, namely:

1. Genes are inherited, but not necessarily the traits associated with them. Environmental factors are necessary for the development of any trait. Theoretically, the expression of *any* gene could be modified by environmental manipulation (though of course most genetic disorders are not as easily remedied as PKU-associated retardation). In a real sense, heredity is *not* destiny.

and

2. The cure for PKU-associated mental retardation most likely would never have been found had the role of the PKU gene not been understood (1996, 86–88, emphasis in original).

An article by Nelkin on the possible (mis)uses of genetic information notes that PKU is a "severe genetic disease that can result in mental retardation" but that it "can be controlled by removing phenylalanine from the diet of afflicted children," and that "[p]ostnatal tests for phenylketonuria . . . have allowed control of this disease through rather simple dietary measures" (1992, 179). Greely, writing on the nearly ubiquitous issue of the Human Genome Project's relationship to health insurance, states that PKU "is a genetic disease that causes severe brain damage, but the damage can be prevented if those affected modify their diets to avoid a certain chemical called phenylalanine" (1992, 272). Dawkins, in the above-quoted letter to *Nature* where he objects to the "suggestion that we are stuck with our biological nature and can't change it," asks that we "recall that warhorse of the genetics textbooks, phenylketonuria" and goes on to mention that this "serious disease, caused by a single recessive gene, is easily cured by rearing the child on a special diet" (1981, 528).[6]

These versions of the story, it seems clear, affirm a form of genetic determinism as well as an emphasis on the genetic and the centrality of the gene. The genetically influenced, in this view, becomes not that which is inevitable or impossible to change, but rather that which can only be avoided or changed through medical, or at least quite deliberate, intervention. In the view that emerges quite naturally from this version of the PKU story, genes do, in fact, determine one's destiny, at least in the absence of clever interventionist doctors (the weak causal version of genetic determinism). And, on this story, it is by attention to the *gene* end of the gene-behavior pathway that we are able to predict, explain, and control those genetically determined problems we would otherwise be stuck with (the methodological stance in favor of the genetic).

A Different Story, and Different Conclusions

But the story as told in the introduction of Plomin et al., and hinted at throughout much of the literature, is at best misleading. Murphey, in his "Phenylketonuria (PKU) and the Single Gene: An Old Story Retold," refers to this story as part of the "scientific and clinical folklore" of human genetics, as a "myth" (1982, 141, 154). Another story, one less bound to this particular myth of PKU as "a winsome example of fact among the largely indecisive findings of behavior genetics" (Murphey 1982, 141),[7] makes the inadequacies of the first story quite clear. Interestingly enough, much of the more sophisticated second story is actually given, albeit rather later, in the Plomin et al. 1990 text, and their own retelling of the story reveals just how misleading was the first story they told.[8]

In the second story (which also has its traditional forms),[9] a dentist with two retarded children is disturbed by the fact that they "exuded a peculiar odor that . . . aggravated his asthmatic condition" (Plomin et al. 1990, 81). He had them examined by Asbjörn Fölling, who, trying to isolate the cause of the odor, found radically elevated levels of phenylpyruvic acid in their urine (this in 1934). From this, Fölling postulated that it was an inborn disturbance in their ability to metabolize phenylalanine that led to the excess of phenylpyruvic acid in their urine and that this was "somehow . . . related to mental retardation" (81). Here the story in Plomin et al. gets condensed somewhat. In Kevles's *In the Name of Eugenics*, we learn of Penroses's early efforts at administering low phenylalanine diets to PKU children almost immediately after Fölling's discoveries (in the mid-1930s) and their failure because those early diets low in phenylalanine were also too low in protein, and resulted in his patients metabolizing their own bodies' proteins, which were not, alas, low in phenylalanine. The extremely high cost of creating wholly synthetic diets low in phenylalanine in the 1930s prevented low-phenylalanine diets from being adequately tested until the 1950s (see Kevles 1985, 177–78).

Here the Plomin text takes up the story again, and makes several interesting points. First, even without dietary therapy, not everyone with one of the genetic defects that causes PKU would suffer the syndrome's many terrible effects. Once PKU screening became easy and potentially useful, it became quite common, and it rapidly became obvious that the assumption that "all phenylketonurics were . . . institutionalized for mental retardation" was false and that many PKU individuals (even those with "classical" high phenylalanine levels in their blood) had IQs solidly in the normal range (Plomin et al. 1990, 82).[10]

A key point to note here is that understanding the gene-behavior pathway had *nothing* to do with the development of the treatment of PKU. Had Fölling *not* hypothesized that it was a single-gene error that prevented phenylalanine from being metabolized (a hypothesis that despite having been widely accepted turned out to be true of only some of the PKU variants; see Murphey 1982), the suggested treatment would have been identical. The move from "excess phenylpyruvic acid" to "inability to metabolize phenylalanine" to "get the phenylalanine out of the diet" has nothing to do with the genetics, nor even the exact biochemical pathways, of the disorder. The problems with the treatment, and their solutions, emerged not from subtle excursions into molecular biology and genetics, but from the sorts of pragmatic (mostly trial-and-error based) medical research that most often advance health care.[11]

The situation, then, was in this case quite the opposite of the known genetics guiding the treatments.[12] Scriver notes that "with hindsight, one sees that the medical phases of PKU history often anticipated its scientific phases" (1995, 137). Indeed, it was the problems with the treatments that gave researchers some of the first hints that the disease might not be as simple as they had thought—that it might be heterogeneous in complex ways (see Murphey 1982, 148, 149). Murphey quotes Reiss, for example, as noting both the presence of clinical and genetic heterogeneity in PKU —clinical heterogeneity in that in different individuals "the same basic defect leads to differing pattern[s] of disease (including normal *mentation*)," and genetic heterogeneity in that several "different genetic factors lead to [a] similar clinical entity" (Reiss, quoted in Murphey 1982, 149, emphasis in original); (see also Hsia 1970). The same gene *for* (genetic defect associated with) PKU can have different results; different genetic defects can (and do) express themselves *as* the clinical condition of PKU.[13] These realizations initially emerged not through any sort of careful genetic studies (linkage, direct sequencing, etc.) but directly from the use of widespread PKU testing, and from those difficulties encountered when children who were thought to have identical conditions reacted very differently to low-phenylalanine diets (there have been accidental retardations and deaths when children without classic PKU were "misdiagnosed" and placed on low-phenylalanine diets) (see Murphey 1982, 149).[14]

Reading the Stories and Recent Twists of the Tale
There are several lessons to be learned from the contrast between these two stories. One is that the claim of understanding a problem because the gene has been found is made in places where it simply isn't the case. The above story makes it clear that "finding the gene" for PKU provided us with almost none of our current understanding of the disease (an understanding that is still far from complete). Another lesson is that the claim is made that cures to diseases follow from finding the gene, or from understanding the genetics, in places where that isn't the case either. "Curing" PKU (preventing retardation) involved trial and error with low-phenylalanine diets (and other biochemical modifications), and the therapy is still developing and advancing. Finding the gene or genes, and indeed, elucidating the heterogeneity of the condition, had (and continues to have) very little to do with treating PKU.[15]

Another point is that even in the absence of medical intervention at the environmental level, the presence of a genetic error correlated with the clinical condition of PKU, even when coupled with the highest diagnostic levels of phenylalanine in the blood, does not guarantee the presence of the classical PKU syndrome (mental retardation). It is not just the possibility of environmental intervention that makes PKU expression nondeterministic; its expression is uncertain in any event.

Indeed, there is currently an interesting war of words in the pediatric-genetics community regarding the clinical heterogeneity of PKU. Some authors currently claim that *any* version of hyperphenylalaninemia that does not result in mental retardation if untreated is, by definition, *not* PKU, but rather non-PKU hyperphenylalaninemia (this is suggested by the American Academy of Pediatrics's Committee on Genetics's "Newborn Screening Fact Sheet" 1996; Eisensmith et al. 1996; and Avigad et al. 1991). The traditional account given in Hsia 1970 makes the diagnosis of "traditional PKU," "nontraditional PKU" and "non-PKU hyperhpenyalaninemia" out to be a matter of blood-serum phenylalanine levels, regardless of whatever effect or lack of one they have on development. While some authors have been so bold as to suggest that all conditions that result from identical mutations in the PAH or BH(4)-coding regions will have the same (or very similar) results (see Eisensmith et al.

1996), this turns out to be false (see Rasmus et al. 1993, Tyfield et al. 1990, and Treacy et al. 1996), so defining PKU by genotype rather than either phenotype at the mentation or phenylalanine blood-serum level does not solve this problem.

Further, many authors currently suggest that a huge percentage of patients with traditional PKU (as measured by blood-serum level) will end up with the traditional PKU syndromes (especially severe mental retardation). The "Newborn Screening Fact Sheet" (1996) claims that some 95 percent of untreated children with traditional PKU will end up with IQs less than 50; Eisensmith et al. claim that "severe, irreversible mental retardation almost always develops" in untreated children with traditional PKU (1996, 513); Vigue, as we saw above, claims that "the symptoms will develop in almost any normal human environments" (1996, 86); Paul claims that "about 90%" of untreated PKU individuals will end up with IQs of less than 50 (1994, 323).[16] What none of these authors give, however, is a citation to any study backing up such numbers; this may have to do with there not having been any such studies. Certainly the limited amount known about the heterogeneity of the clinical manifestations of given mutations would not point toward any such numbers (see Rasmus et al. 1993, Tyfield et al. 1990), and the initial study of treated versus untreated siblings that Berman et al. published in 1969 would not point toward such high percentages. Of course, for all that is currently known, the figure of 95 percent could be accurate; after all, nothing is known about the genotypes of Berman's PKU patients, and studies such as Rasmus's are too small to be statistically significant. Then again, such high numbers could just as easily be wildly misleading. Indeed, based on Berman et al. 1969 and the smaller studies, one could be forgiven for thinking that such high figures probably *are* misleading. It is the very good fortune of PKU individuals that screening and treatment in the developed world is nearly universal (which is not to say that more research on diet, better diagnostic tools, etc., are not still needed; see Scriver 1995); it is, however, unfortunate for those who wish to know what percentage of PKU individuals would have normal development without intervention. Given that tradeoff, this is an ignorance I think we can well live with. However, researchers would do well to admit that we have no idea what percentage of individuals with mutations associated with PKU would have normal intellectual functioning without intervention, rather than citing numbers that seem at best dubious. And we might well ask why, given the lack of data and the uncertainty, such a high number is cited. It does not seem unreasonable to argue that the habit of thinking of gene-phenotype pathways as "nearly certain" in the absence of intervention has something to do with this.

As a last point, I'd like to stress that the Plomin et al. 1990 text is not interesting because it underestimates the complexities of PKU, but rather because, unlike most pieces on the subject, it eventually gets around to telling a more complete story. The way this happens, with the myth serving as a warning about the falsity of genetic determinism in the introduction, followed by the actual history tucked into a chapter on the "Mechanisms of Heredity and Behavior," brings out another point. Even researchers in human genetics who are careful about historical details tend to vastly overestimate the importance of the genetics when they aren't being quite as careful, and they do so in ways that make the genetics seem much more central, much more practical, and much more deterministic than their more careful stories would allow for.

The first of the PKU stories, then, the "mythical PKU," should be read not as a warning about the limits of genetic determinism but rather as pointing toward the sort of genetic determinism that many researchers implicitly believe in, and indeed take for granted. That such a story, with its emphasis on the genetic as central to prediction and control of behavior, and its hints of near-certain gene-behavior pathways, can be turned into a warning about the limits of genetic determinism reveals what a radical version of genetic determinism the researchers stand against when they claim to stand against the thesis. In opposing one form of genetic determinism, then, another form— one that is both subtler and more insidious—gets slipped in, completely without argument.

In the next chapter we will see how this and similar convictions in the certainty of causal pathways and the ease of understanding them result in the power of various techniques to study the relationship between genetics and complex human traits being systematically overestimated. The argument, again, will not be that it is impossible that the relationships argued for really exist, but rather that the research that purports to support such relationships fails to do so.

CHAPTER 3

GENES AND CAUSATION

Techniques for Explaining Differences

If it were possible to accurately model the development of arbitrarily complex organisms from fertilized eggs to their adult forms at arbitrary levels of detail, questions about the relative importance of genes, environments, and genotype-environment interactions would probably seem much less pressing. Indeed, since it is obvious that at each stage of the modeling process imagined the development of the organism would depend on all these factors and the complex relationships among them, the question might appear entirely moot. While it is likely that for certain classes of organisms (for example, fruit flies, flatworms) developmental biology may eventually come close to achieving this goal, it is also possible that the world is not deterministic and mathematically/physically tractable enough to permit such a modeling in the case of mammals and other very complex organisms (see Dupré 1993). At the very least, models that deal with the developmental biology of arbitrarily complex organisms by tracing low-level biochemical and biophysical paths from genes to phenotypes during development in specific environments are promises for the far, distant future.

Given this limitation, it is often thought that in explaining those differences that matter to us in humans we must make use of techniques that are rather less exacting than the full developmental approach suggested above. The primary focus of this chapter is on those techniques that are used in research projects that focus on trying to explain differences between humans as somehow related to genetic differences. In discussing the various techniques employed (and to which reference is made in published works and public discussions) the concern will be to bring out the strengths and limitations of the various techniques with respect to their use in explaining differences between humans for the interestingly complex traits that we care about. Some of these techniques have other uses (many of which are also well established) within various other domains, and certainly some of the criticisms made of their use in, for example, human behavior genetics would be inappropriate if generalized to encompass all their possible and actual uses.

While I will for the most part be discussing the techniques used in exploring the relationship between genetic differences among individuals and differences in complex traits as if they were separate, it should be kept in mind that for any particular trait, researchers who work on trying to discover possible genetic causes and give explanations of differences in that trait often attempt to apply many different techniques to the particular problem they are interested in. So, for example, in thinking about the possible genetic etiology for mood-affective disorders, as we shall see, researchers bring in estimates of heritability, molecular genetics findings, and evolutionary reasoning in order to attempt to support their arguments. A brief example of this is presented below, where evolutionary reasoning is seen combined with molecular genetics findings and heritability estimates in explaining variation in "novelty seeking" in humans. More generally, though, how these techniques are meant to relate to each other will be brought up briefly within the individual discussions of the techniques and then more thoroughly in the individual cases to which they are applied in later chapters.

Heritability: What It Is, What It (Doesn't) Mean, and Why It Won't Just Go Away

Since it is currently impossible to simultaneously model all the relevant developmental pathways in complex organisms, and many questions about the details of human evolution remain unanswered, questions about the relative importance of genes and environments to traits that vary quantitatively within given populations are often still considered relevant. This is of course a very different question than that which the strict developmental approach hinted at above would answer, and it is important to realize that the answers don't (can't) do the same "work." One must take care not to confuse the answers to the one sort of question with the answers to the other; all too often, though, such care isn't taken. In any event, pretty much everyone currently admits that every phenotypic trait is the result of the interaction of both genes and the environment (see Kitcher 1999 for a discussion of the ubiquity of the "interactionist" thesis). Further, it is obviously senseless to ask what percentage of any given trait is owed to genes or environment *simpliciter* (see Lewontin 1974, 110). To take a common example, height, the idea is that we cannot ask of a person who is, say, 62 inches tall, what fraction of those 62 inches come from genes and what fraction from the environment. Obviously, both genes and environment were necessary for the person's height—for them to have any height to measure at all!—and there is no way of dividing up the total.

What *is* often asked in place of this is what percentage of the *variation* of particular phenotypic traits within a population is attributable to genetic or environmental variation. For a population with an average height of, say, 58 inches, the question that is often raised is how much of the *differences* from these 58 inches are the results of differences in the genetic makeup of the population and how much are the results of differences in the environments (developmental and otherwise) of the population. *Broad-sense heritability* (often referred to simply as *heritability* in the literature on human behavior genetics) is the proportion of phenotypic variance (*variance*, the squared difference from the mean, is used rather than the difference from the mean *simpliciter* for technical reasons) in a population that is "attributable" to that population's genetic variation;[1] *environmentality* (a term suggested by Plomin et al. 1990 as the complementary concept to broad-sense heritability) is the percentage of phenotypic variance in a population that is "attributable" to environmental variation. I make many simplifying assumptions below in discussing analysis of variance as given by the standard models in quantitative genetics. However, these assumptions in no way influence any of the critiques of the use of, for example, estimates of heritability in human populations (see box 3.1).

The "standard equation" for analyzing the variance in phenotypic differences is

$$P = G + E + GE + e$$

where P is the total phenotypic variance in the population, G is the variance shared by those members of the population who share the relevant genotype, E is the variance shared by those members who share the relevant environment, GE is the variance shared by those members who share both the relevant genotype and the relevant environment but which is not simply the additive effects of G and E (it is often referred to as the gene-environment interaction term), and "e" is everything else.[2] Heritability, then, is:

$$H^2 = G / P$$

If you know the heritability of a trait within a population, just what is it that you know? What predictions are you justified in making? Over the years, many claims have been made about what the high heritability of some given trait in some population "means" for understanding the trait, making predictions about the trait, or even for social policy. While the individual chapters give a better sense of the extent and character of these claims, I'd like to give a few examples here just to get the flavor of these kinds of claims. So, for example, Jung claims that the high heritability of obesity "removes this condition from a social stigma to the disease category" and implies that it is "an actual disease" (1997, 307). Hamer and Copeland take the high heritability of IQ scores to mean that "no other single factor is more important than genes in determining cognitive ability" (1998, 219). Hamer and Copeland go on to claim that the very high heritability (they give a figure of "70 to 90 percent") of very shy or inhibited personality types is "probably the reason it doesn't change much during a lifetime" (1998, 66–67). Famously, Murray and Herrnstein argued that the high heritability of IQ meant that, in a society that sorted itself according to ability, some people were going to be stuck at the bottom because of inherited differences, and nothing much could or should be done about this (see Murray and Herrnstein 1994, 105; see also Jensen 1969). Kendler argues that the frequency of "stressful life events" encountered is "genetically influenced" through the high heritability of temperament, and that this means that it is "because of differences in genetic constitution" that people "select themselves into high versus low risk environments" (1998, 8). DiLalla and Gottesman argued from the high heritability of "anti-social behavior" to the conclusion that understanding "intergenerational transmission" of violence and abusive behavior will require understanding the "genetic and biological factors" which "influence violent crime" and that "social policy decisions" formed without such an understanding will likely be "faulty" (1991, 128). Judge Parslow, deciding a famous custody battle in California, cited the high heritability of IQ and other behavioral traits as a reason why genetic parenthood should determine custody; paradoxically, Annas argued from the high heritability of IQ to the conclusion that a child's "best interests" might not be served by giving custody to his or her genetic parents, since he or she would probably do about the same in life whatever the environment s/he ends up in (see Superior Court of Orange County, Nos. X-633190 and AD-57638 at 7, Annas 1991; this case is discussed in chapter 9; see also Krim 1996 for discussion). In other cases of legal actions, the high

Box 3.1: Calculating Heritability: An Example

If the *variance* of a trait (the average squared deviation from the population mean) within a population (P) is accounted for by reference to the phenotypic variance of that trait in the population that is shared by those members of the population that share relevant genotypes (G), the phenotypic variance of that trait in the population that is shared by those members of the population that share relevant environments (E), and the phenotypic variance that is shared by those members of the population that share both relevant genotypes and environments but cannot be accounted for by the additive effects of G and E (GE), and "everything else" (including random developmental noise, error, etc.), then:

$$P = G + E + GE + e$$

where organisms with particular genotypes are spread throughout the relevant environments in a random way (where there is no correlation between an organism's possessing a particular genotype and developing in a particular environments; see note 2,).

Given this, the broad-sense heritability (H^2) of a trait within a population is defined as the fraction of the phenotypic variance in the population shared by those members of the population that share relevant genotypes:

$$H^2 = G / P$$

Consider the following example, adapted from Cooper and Zubek's (1958) work on maze-running ability in rats. Consider a population consisting of six individuals and three environments. Individuals are either genotype G(A) or G(B); environments are either type E(1), E(2), or E(3). One individual of each genotype appears in each environment; the measured phenotypes for each genotype in each environment is as follows:

	G(A)	G(B)
E(1)	170	170
E(2)	117	164
E(3)	111	120

The phenotypic average for the population is 142; the *variance* of trait in this population (the average squared deviation from the mean) is 687 squared units. The average variance shared by those organisms that share a relevant genotype (G(A) or G(B)) is about 87.11 squared units.

Heritability (H^2) is therefore 87.11 / 687, or .127

The average variance shared by those organisms that share relevant environments (1, 2, or 3) is about 496 squared units, so environmentality, or the fraction of the total phenotypic variance shared by those organisms that share relevant environments (1, 2, or 3), will be about .72.

heritability of IQ has been used to justify testing the intelligence of parents and other relatives in cases involving liability for lead poisoning; the theory, apparently, is that if the parents aren't too bright, and IQ is heritable, then the lead probably wasn't at fault for the child's problems after all (see Wriggins 1997).

Despite the many calls that have been made over the years for scientists to stop spending their time trying to calculate broad-sense heritability for traits in humans, and for people to stop publishing research based on it (see Lewontin 1974; Feldman and Lewontin 1975; Oyama 1985; Block 1995; Kitcher 1999), researchers have obviously neither stopped working to calculate it nor to interpret it. Nor are these interpretations "trivial" ones that don't influence policy or people's lives—rather, they go to the heart of our conceptions of ourselves and influence policies and legal decisions that affect some of the most important aspects of our lives.

However, the above claims about what knowing the high heritability of a trait tells us—what it is possible to change, what kinds of features are "real," what "social policies" would be advisable, and the like—are, quite simply, unfounded. This is the reason why various authors have called, albeit with little success, for people to stop using and to stop trying to estimate the heritability of traits in human populations. The claims are wrong for technical reasons, and are entirely insupportable without the addition of a number of very questionable assumptions—assumptions for which, I argue, we have no evidence nor any way of gathering evidence. It is unfortunate that even where other methods that are generally considered more "direct" (for example, molecular methods) are beginning to generate some results in human cases, many studies are still centered on measures of heritability, and other studies supplement molecular-level findings with estimates of heritability (see the chapters on specific cases for examples). And, as the uses of heritability cited above suggested, many researchers still claim that such estimates are useful.[3] For this reason I think it is worth trying to bring out the limitations of the concept of heritability yet again.

Heritability estimates in human populations suffer from another major limitation as well. Generating an accurate estimate of the heritability of a trait in a natural population is fiendishly difficult; indeed, some recent arguments have been put forward that it is in principle impossible to generate accurate heritability estimates except in populations where one has access to controlled breeding and controlled environments (see Bailey 1997). Obviously, human populations will provide particular challenges here. This problem is, in some ways, less serious than the conceptional limitations of heritability. It isn't a limitation on what, in principle, the heritability of a trait in a population can be used to explain or predict, but rather a limitation on how seriously we should take the estimates that are given by various research groups and reported in the popular press. However, if the conceptual limitations are taken as seriously as I believe they should be, this limitation will seem fairly pointless—it doesn't matter how good or bad an estimate of heritability you have if that estimate is of no use for making the sorts of predictions you wish to make, or for explaining the sorts of things you wish to use it to explain.

What Does "Heritability" Mean?

Heritability is usually given one of two interpretations. However, both of them are problematic. Here the two interpretations are presented, and some of the problems with these interpretations discussed.

On one interpretation of broad-sense heritability (H^2), it is the proportion of the variance of the phenotype in question in the population in question that is "attributable" to genetic differences within that population. Crow calls this the "variance," or "population," interpretation (see Crow 1986). This is the interpretation most naturally suggested by the presentation of the basic equations used to think through analysis of variance (see above), and it is worth going through an example that displays this interpretation. Crow discusses Wright's experiments with spotted guinea pigs. He notes that for the trait "degree of white spotting," given a total variance in the population of 573 squared units,[4] and a broad-sense heritability of about .4, the population interpretation claims that about .4 of the total variance in that population—that is, about 229 squared units—is "attributable" to the genetic variation, and some 344 squared units are "attributable" to the environmental variation (Crow 1986, 126). Plomin et al. follow this interpretation at times. For example, in their discussion of heritability book's in the appendix, they state that a heritability of .5 means that "50 percent of the phenotypic variance is explained by genetic variance . . . the other 50 percent . . . is caused by environmental variance" (Plomin et al. 1997, 300).

Occasionally, this is taken to mean that if the genotypic variation were eliminated, all the variance "attributed" to genetic variation would be eliminated; that is, in Wright's example, that 229 squared units of the variation would be eliminated, and the total variation would be reduced to 344 squared units. Alternately, it is suggested that eliminating environmental variation would reduce the total phenotypic variation to the 229 squared units "attributable" to genetic variation. And, indeed, when Crow states that

> [i]f all the individuals could be reared in identical environments, the phenotypic variance, V_P, would be reduced to V_H [variance shared by those

organisms that share the same relevant genotype — written "G" above].
Alternately if the individuals were all of the same genotype, the variance
would reduce to V_E" (Crow 1986, 126),

it certainly seems to suggest such an interpretation, as does the notion of
the squared units of variation being "attributable" to genetic or environmental variation respectively. However, this particular way of looking at
the population interpretation should be resisted, as it is at best very misleading. Depending on the way in which genotypic or environmental
variation is eliminated, total phenotypic variance can, far from being
reduced as the above suggests, actually be *increased*. Essentially, this is
because different genotypes are differentially sensitive to differences in
environments, and if, for example, all the genotypes but the most sensitive
are eliminated, total phenotypic variation may actually be increased.

Consider the following example, adapted from Cooper and Zubek's
work on breeding rats for "maze-running ability" (1958).[5] Cooper and
Zubek started with two strains of rats that had been selected, in a "normal" laboratory environment, to be either very good at running mazes or
very bad at it; these were called "maze-bright" rats and "maze-dull" rats,
respectively. When reared in the normal environment, "maze-bright" rats
made relatively few errors running mazes (around 117 errors), and "maze-
dull" rats made relatively many errors (around 164). Cooper and Zubek
then raised these two strains of rats in other environments and tested
their maze-running ability. In an "enriched" environment, an environment with lots of toys and visual stimulation, bright rats made around 111
errors, and dull rats made around 120 errors. This difference, 111 errors
versus 120 errors, was not statistically significant. In a "restricted" environment; that is, an environment with gray cages and no moving parts,
both strains of rats made around 170 errors (Cooper and Zubek 1958).

One way to display this information is with a *reaction norm*, the graph
that results when organisms of a given relevant genotype are raised in several different environments and the resulting phenotype is plotted. Here,
one is plotting the average numbers of errors made in each of three environments for each of the two strains of rat (see figure 3.1).[6]

Consider a population consisting of rats of both types, with equal numbers in each environment. It is clear that in this situation one would measure some heritability of maze-running ability, since maze-bright rats do
better on average than maze-dull rats. It is clear as well that there is also an
environmental component to maze-running ability, since rats reared in an
enriched environment do better on average than those reared in a
restricted or normal environment (see figure 3.1 and box 3.1). What hap-

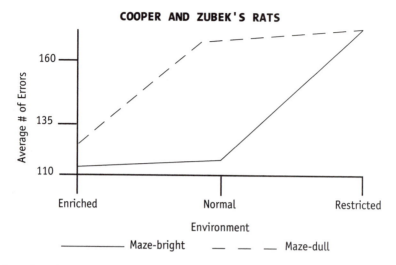

Data for Figure 3.1

Average number of errors made for two types of rats in three environments:

Environment/Rat Type	Enriched	Normal	Restricted
Maze-bright	111.2	117	169.7
Maze-dull	119.7	164	169.5

Figure 3.1: Cooper and Zubek's Rats. Cooper and Zubek (1958) began their research with two strains of rats. These strains had been bred (by McGill) from an original stock to be either very good ("maze-bright") or very bad ("maze-dull") at running mazes. The selection was done in a "normal" laboratory environment. When Cooper and Zubek worked with the rats that were raised under ordinary laboratory conditions (the "normal" environment), the maze-bright rats significantly outperformed (made far fewer errors then) the maze-dull rats.

However, when the environment in which the rats were raised was replaced with either an "enriched" environment (one with lots of toys, etc.) or an "impoverished" environment (gray cages with no movable objects), there was no longer any statistically significant difference between the strains. In the enriched environment, both performed very well; in the impoverished environment, both strains performed very poorly.

This can be seen on a reaction norm, in which the "ecotype" (an ecotype is a population that has undergone selection in a particular environment and become adapted to that environment—in this case, two ecotypes resulted from the different selective pressures the two strains faced) is plotted against the environmental variable.

Notice that the maze-bright rats only outperform the maze-dull rats in one of the three environments tested.

pens, though, if we eliminate all the environment variation? Will phenotypic variance be reduced, as the interpretation given by Crow suggests?

It should be clear that this depends completely on *how* we reduce the environmental variation (see box 3.2). If we eliminate enriched and normal environments, leaving only the restricted environment, we would indeed reduce the phenotypic variance; in fact, we would eliminate *all* the variation. This is rather more than the interpretation given by Crow would have suggested! On the other hand, if we eliminate the enriched and restricted environments and leave only the normal environment, the total variance of the population would actually *increase*, since it is only in that environment that there are large average deviations from the mean.

The other interpretation often given to estimates of broad-sense heritability is the "individual" interpretation. In this interpretation, the claim is that the difference in the phenotypic value in some trait of an individual from the population mean is to be accounted for by reference to the

---

Box 3.2: Reaction Norms and Heritability

Consider the reaction norm for "maze-bright" and "maze-dull" rats in the three environments Cooper and Zubek tested them. (see figure 3.1) As we saw in box 3.1, in a mixed population of roughly equal numbers of maze-bright and maze-dull rats, with equal numbers of rats raised in each of the three environments, a large component of the variation from the average maze-running ability will be accountable for by environmental variation (because, on average, the better environments yield lower error scores), and a substantial component will be accounted for by genetic variation (since, on average, maze-bright rats score better than maze-dull rats). Hence, there is both substantial *environmentality* and substantial *heritability*.

However, what happens if no rats are raised in the "normal" environment? Notice that the genetic component to the variations *vanishes*, since there is no significant difference in performance between maze-bright and maze-dull rats in either "enriched" or "restricted" environments (the only two left).

On the other hand, raising most or all of the rats in the "normal" environment, and very few or none in the enriched and restricted environments, would have the effect of *increasing* both the total phenotypic variance of the population, and also increasing the heritability of maze-running ability, as more of the variation in the population would be correlated with genetic variation and less with environmental variation. As the number of rats in the restricted and enriched environments went to zero, the heritability of maze-running ability in the population would go to one.

The upshot is that neither a very low, nor a very high, heritability for a trait can be used to argue that environmental changes would be ineffective in changing the phenotypes of the organisms!

heritability and environmentality of that trait within the population. Crow and Plomin et al. give the identical example of a man who is "10 inches above the average" where the heritability of height in the population is .8. Crow states that such a man "can attribute 8 of the 10 inches by which he exceeds the population average to his genotype and the other 2 inches to his environment" (Crow 1986, 126–27; Plomin et al. 1990, 232). While again it is generally agreed to be senseless to ask of a man who is, say, 72 inches tall what percentage of his height he owes to his environment and what to his genotype, the idea is that it is sensible to ask what proportion of his *difference* from the population mean can be accounted for by his environment and what proportion by his genotype. Plomin et al. consider that this estimate is "rather imprecise" (1990, 232),[7] and Crow notes that it is "based on averages" and that "individual values differ widely" (1986, 126–27); both, however, seem to take this interpretation seriously.

Whether this interpretation *should* be taken seriously is actually a fairly deep problem. To follow the examples of Crow and Plomin et al. we might (perhaps naively) expect that a large number of men who are 10 inches above the average height would, if raised in an average environment, have their average height reduced by some 2 inches.[8] However, when applied to a single individual, there is some reason to doubt that this claim can be defended.

Crow claims that for an individual with a larger than average phenotypic value (such as height in this example), "usually" both genetic and environmental "influences are involved" such that "part of the excess height is caused by the genotype and part by the environment" (1986, 125). Prima facie, there seems to be no reason to expect that an individual with a genotype that in a given population and a given distribution of environments would favor a higher than average height would also tend to be reared in an environment that would favor such a height advantage as well. Of course, for some traits where differences from the mean are influenced by both environmental and genetic differences, these differences might in fact covary positively. But, of course, some don't covary at all, and even among those that do, the direction in which they covary is not a given. Without additional information about the way that G and E covary within the given population, there seems to be no reason to suspect that a person with a genotype that tends to result in higher than average phenotypic values within a population will tend to have a higher than average chance of being reared in environments with that feature as well.[9]

Perhaps more to the point, such an interpretation would yield simply ludicrous results in some cases. Recalling that the difference in numbers of errors made by Cooper and Zubek's maze-bight and maze-dull rats in the enriched and restricted environments was not judged statistically significant (Cooper and Zubek 1958, 160–61), we can consider a simplified norm of reaction for the maze-bright and maze-dull rats in restricted and normal environments only where only statistically significant differences are shown (see figure 3.2). Again, notice that there is both a positive heritability and a positive "environmentality" in this example.[10] Here, if we followed Plomin et al. (1990) and Crow on the individual interpretation of heritability, we would be forced to say that, for example, rats that made relatively many errors owe some of that lack of ability to being in a worse environment, and some to having a worse genotype. But in this case, that is simply *false*. The number of errors that maze-dull rats make is essentially *independent* of whether they are in the restricted or the normal environment, as there is no significant difference in the error rates for maze-dull rats between restricted and normal environments.

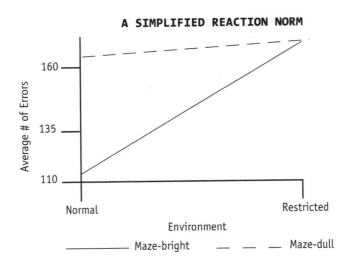

A SIMPLIFIED REACTION NORM

Average # of Errors

Environment

——————— Maze-bright   — — — Maze-dull

Data for Figure 3.2

Average number of errors made for two types of rats in two types of environments:

Environment/Rat Type	Normal	Restricted
Maze-Bright	117	169.7
Maze-dull	164	169.5

Figure 3.2: A simplified reaction norm. Notice that the number of errors (about 170) made by "maze-dull" rats is essentially independent of whether they are in the normal or the restricted environment.

Neither of the two common interpretations given to heritability seem particularly satisfying, then. How serious a problem this is, given that in human behavior genetics heritability is usually not given any interpretation at all, is an open question. However, the difficulties encountered in trying to make sense of the two interpretations usually given hint at more serious conceptual problems and limitations of the concept.

Estimating Heritability

Before discussing the most serious conceptual flaws with the concept of heritability, it is worth mentioning just how difficult it is to generate reliable and convincing estimates of the heritability of complex traits, or indeed even simple traits, in humans. To estimate the heritability of a trait, the basic trick is to disentangle the environmental effects from the genetic effects. The best way to do this is to distribute organisms with known genotypes into controlled environments and see what happens. When one is using experimental animals or plants, one can simply distribute genetically identical, or relevantly similar, animals into the environments to be tested in a systematic way. The most striking form of this approach is where *clones*, genetically identical animals, are distributed into the same range of environments as the population generally. Since the gestational environment sometimes matters to the trait in question, a confounding factor is that part of the environment of clones gestated in vivo is shared, no matter how soon after birth the organisms are randomized. To get around this problem the clones can be generated in vitro and the randomizing done at their implantation. Using this method, it is, at least in principle, possible to calculate the broad-sense heritability of the trait in question directly from any correlations in the trait shared only by the genetic clones. The amount that differences in the trait in question shared by the clones is systematically different from the average amount that the trait in question varies within the population provides a fairly direct estimate of heritability.[11] Other methods used with lab animals are less satisfactory, but the basic idea—to randomize individuals with respect to their genes and their environment—is the same (these methods are discussed in Plomin et al. 1990).[12]

Since researchers interested in estimating the heritability of complex traits in humans cannot control the environments or the breeding of their experimental subjects, various techniques must be used to try to get around these limitations. Again, the basic technique is to use some analysis of covariance among genetically related individuals and then to somehow try to control for the possibility of shared environmental influences.

The most convincing estimates of the broad-sense heritability of complex behavioral traits in humans—or other kinds of traits, for that matter—

would come from showing correlations in the phenotypic variation of genetically identical people who had no environmental correlations at all during development, over and above those shared by genetically unrelated individuals (see Lewontin et al. 1984, 101ff.; and Plomin et al. 1990, 346–47). This would be the equivalent of those heritability estimates discussed above, performed on experimental animals using clones and deliberately randomized environments. The closest thing to this with humans is monozygotic (identical) twins who were separated at birth and raised apart. If one wanted really convincing evidence, of course, one would start with large numbers of genetically identical embryos and separate them well *before* birth, in order to remove any influence the gestational environment might have. That is, one would take care to implant the embryos in uncorrelated gestational environments in order to ensure that gestational environments were not influencing the results, and one would start with large numbers in order to generate sample sizes that would be statistically significant. With humans, of course, such techniques are out of the question. The impossibility of doing experiments of that sort already puts limitations on the accuracy of any technique based on "separated twins." The effects of shared gestational environments should not be thought trivial. Recent work on the effects of the prenatal environment point toward its having large phenotypic consequences. Further, the fact that most monozygotic but not dizygotic ("fraternal") twins share a placenta is thought to be a possible explanation for at least some of the extra covariance in monozygotic twins as compared to dizygotic twins (see for example Davis et al. 1995; Machin 1996; Gottlieb and Manchester 1986; for a quick survey, see also *"Double Trouble,"* Nov. 18 1995, 89–91).

Alternately, rather than hoping to find rather rare, and perhaps mostly mythical twins separated at birth and raised in uncorrelated environments, (see Horgan 1993 and Lewontin et al. 1984) "normal" adoptions can be used to try to ferret out some of the effects of the environment. By comparing, for example, the phenotypic correlations of full siblings adopted apart, half siblings adopted apart, biological parents and their adopted-away offspring, adoptive parents and their unrelated offspring, and genetically unrelated adoptive siblings (genetically unrelated individuals adopted together), different estimates of heritability can be generated. In each case there are difficulties with the estimates, but taken together they are thought to provide a rough picture of broad-sense heritability. While it is impossible to fully separate out genetic differences from environmental differences using these methods, it is thought that with enough different kinds of data, some plausible estimates of broad-sense heritability can be made.

At least, it is thought, such methods yield more reliable results than any single kind of data, or than just guessing. One problem with these methods has traditionally been the phenomena of selective placement. Adoption agencies often attempt to place children in homes more like the homes of their biological parents than chance alone would yield (see Lewontin et al. 1984). Selective placement—that is, placement that tends to match adopted children to adoptive parents with respect to race, religion, or other cultural factors—is a serious problem for studies of separated twins as well. In any event, selective placement makes untangling the environmental and genetic influences much more difficult, if not impossible. Another problem is the inability of such methods to fully account for non-additive genetic effects (see above and Plomin et al. 1990 for details). Even so, it is hoped that differences between the correlations in full siblings and those between parents and their offspring or half siblings can be used to extract some information about the effects of dominance; that differences between the regressions of unrelated offspring toward their adoptive parents and the regressions of offspring toward those genetically related parents who raised them, as well as the differences in correlations between unrelated adoptive siblings and genetically related siblings, can provide some estimates of the effects of shared environments, and the like.

Studies of the sort described above, so-called full adoption studies, are somewhat complex, as they require many sorts of relationships to be tracked over adoptions. Further, those studies that have been done have tended to generate surprising numbers of rather odd results along with those results that might be expected, and that tend to be prominently featured in the research reports and media coverage (see Lewontin et al. 1984). For example, *some* of the results of the Texas Adoption Project, which is often thought of as being a particularly good example of a full adoption study, are cited relatively often (see Plomin et al. 1990, for example). An example of a result that is easily explained and cited fairly often is the finding that the correlation between the adoptive parents' IQs and those of the adopted children were low, less than half that of the adopted children and their genetic parents. This, it is argued, points toward the genetic relationship's being important. However, it is more rarely mentioned that the IQs of the adoptive parents in this study were not highly correlated with *their own* genetic children either; indeed, the correlations are no higher than those they share with their adopted children (see Horn et al. 1979, 192)! Neither is it usually mentioned that on some of the tests the Texas Adoption Project used, the genetic mothers of adopted away children had significant correlations with *other* children adopted into the same family—children with whom they shared *neither* genes *nor* an environment (see Horn et al. 1979, 208, table 1). These correlations were higher than, for example, those that the adoptive parents had with *their own* genetic children, with whom they shared *both* genes and environment! I suggest that such bizarre results undermine the simplistic interpretations given to those results that are more easily explained.

Another technique for attempting to tease apart the effects of the environment and genes is to look at the correlations of monozygotic twins reared together and the correlations of dizygotic but same-sex twins, again reared together. The key assumption in this sort of study is that twins of either sort, when raised in the same family, will share familial environments to about the same extent, and so shared environmental influences should be the same for both sorts of twins. This is a substantive and contestable assumption for several reasons. One of them, discussed above, is that (most) monozygotic twins share a placenta, and so have a more similar gestational environment than do dizygotic twins, most of whom do not share a placenta. Another is that the environments of identical twins are different in important ways from those of dizygotic twins. In any event, since monozygotic twins share all their genetic influences, and dizygotic twins only those that ordinary full siblings would share, it is argued that the amount that the covariances of monozygotic and dizygotic twins differ can yield an estimate of the extent of the genetic influences (see for example Plomin et al. 1990, 1997). However, it is impossible to accurately account for the different effects of nonadditive genetic influences using these methods, so their results are always somewhat contestable (nonadditive genetic influences are related to such phenomena as dominance, epistasis, and genetic covariances, which are discussed below).

None of these techniques are able to account for the possibility of complex interactions between genes and their context. Bailey, for example, argues that even under ideal conditions of twins separated at birth, the inability to truly randomize environments means that possible covariances between genes and environments make heritability estimates questionable. These covariances could be caused by, for example, an individual's ability to self-select environments. Further, Bailey notes that the possibility of complex (e.g., nonlinear) interactions between genes and environments further undermines the reliability of heritability estimates in human populations. In fact, Bailey goes somewhat beyond this claim to note that "even *qualitative* statements about the relative role of genes and the environment in affecting behavior and cognitive ability (e.g., Plomin et al. 1994) are foolhardy" (Bailey 1997, 129, emphasis added).[13] Insofar as we suspect that complex human traits at least may involve such complex interactions among genes, suites of genes, and their contexts, it is hard to have much confidence in the estimates of heritability often cited.

Be that as it may, the accuracy of estimates of heritability really aren't the issue at all in thinking about their use in human behavior genetics, as I hope the next section will make clear. The conceptual problems with heritability estimates, no matter how accurate they may be, make them useless for explaining differences in traits that we care about in people (e.g., intelligence, obesity, depression, alcoholism, violence, etc.), or for predicting how various kinds of policy decisions could change the distributions of those traits in the population.

Conceptual Limitations of Heritability: Differences and Locality
It has long been recognized that there are serious limitations to the usefulness of the concept of broad-sense heritability when thinking about human populations. The most important limitation is a conceptual one: heritability is a local measure. The main point of this section will be to explore what it means to say that heritability is a local measure and why this matters. Briefly, by "local measure" I mean a measure that depends in large part on contingent features of the population in question; that is, it is a measure that depends upon features of the population that can, and often do, change over time (this definition, and much of the following discussion, follows Lewontin 1974). The broad-sense heritability of a trait within a population depends on the current genetic makeup of the population, the current environment(s) that the population finds itself in, and the way various member organisms of the population are distributed within these environments. Change any of these things and the heritability of the trait in question can, and often does, change as well.

For this reason, heritability alone is not a useful feature of a population for thinking about what kinds of effects changes will make in the population. In other words knowing the heritability of a trait within a population will not permit you to make predictions about what will happen if changes occur in either the environment, the genetic distributions, or the way that the population is distributed with respect to the environment. In human populations, where often all that can be given is an estimate of the heritability of some trait, attempts to use this number in formulating social policy will clearly be shown to be misguided.

EXAMPLES OF LOCALITY[14] Again, to say that heritability is a local measure is just to point out that it "depends upon the actual distribution of genotypes and environments in the particular population sampled" (Lewontin 1974, 113). If any of these contingent facts change, the heritability may change as well (see below and box 3.3). More to the point,

---

Box 3.3: The Locality of Heritability

As Lewontin noted in his 1974 article "The Analysis of Variance and the Analysis of Causes," broad-sense heritability is a *local* measure. Heritability depends upon characteristics of populations that can and do change. Some examples of characteristics that can change and could influence the measured heritability of a trait include:

1) The distribution of organisms into environments

   a) Available environments can be encountered with different frequencies by the population in general.

   b) Organisms may change the way they are distributed into the available environments by, for example, sorting themselves into different environments *depending on their relevant genetic makeup.*

2) The environments available

   a) If some environments simply become more common, then the organisms in the population may well sort themselves into the available environments differently.

   b) If the range of available environments is either reduced (some environments no longer exist) or is increased (some new environments come into existence), then organisms in the population may well end up in different relevant environments.

3) The distribution of relevantly similar types of organisms in the population

   a) The proportion of organisms of a particular type may change.

4) The relevantly similar types of organisms available

   a) The range of types of organisms in a population may be increased—that is, new, and relevantly different, types of organisms may become available in the population. Or the range of types of organisms in a population may be decreased—that is, the frequency of a particular type of organism in a population may drop to zero.

---

without making some very strong, and indeed implausible, assumptions, estimates of heritability cannot be used to predict what effects changing the environment might have on the population in question, nor can they be used to explain the relationship between the environment, the contemporary population, and the trait in question.

Consider again Cooper and Zubek's study of maze-bright and maze-dull rats. One way that has already been hinted at of changing the heritability of maze-running ability would be to change the distribution of the organisms within the three possible environments. If far more rats of each type were in the "normal" environment than in either the "enriched" or the "restricted" environments, heritability would be higher; indeed, heritability would tend toward 100 percent as the percentage of rats in the normal environment went toward 100. However, if far more rats of each type were in the enriched or restricted environments, heritability would be lower; under these conditions, heritability would tend toward zero as the percentage of rats in the normal environment went toward zero. These, in general, can be thought of as changes in the *distribution* of organisms into environments. So if all we knew of a population of Cooper and Zubek's rats was that the heritability was 100 percent, would this allow us to predict anything about how the phenotypes would react to different environments? Clearly not. Would it tell us anything about how easy or difficult the traits would be to change through environmental interventions? It would not. High heritability alone does not countenance those sorts of claims.

Another way of changing the distribution of organisms into environments is to permit the types of organisms—relevantly similar genotypes—to sort themselves into different environments in a nonrandom way. Permitting the type of organism to *covary* with the type of environment makes calculating broad-sense heritability rather trickier; in any event, it will clearly change it. Imagine, in the original Cooper and Zubek example (figure 3.1), if all the maze-bright rats tended to stay in restricted environments and all the maze-dull rats tended to stay in the enriched environments. In such a situation, heritability would cease to be even a coherent measure in the population!

Another way of changing heritability is to change the types of environments available. If the maze-running experiment had been done with *only* restricted and enriched environments, heritability would naturally be quite low; if a normal environment were then added, heritability would increase. Similarly, of course, if we simply eliminated the normal environment from our original example, we would decrease heritability. Changes of this sort can be thought of as changes in the *range* of environments available.

Yet another kind of change can occur when the proportion of a particular genotype changes in a population. So, considering our simplified two-environment example again, if we increased the proportion of maze-dull rats, the heritability of maze-running ability will actually increase.

This is because maze-dull rats are relatively unaffected by the environmental variation in this example. These changes might be called changes in the genotypic *frequencies.*

For the next kind of possible change, a hypothetical organism will be introduced. Call it the "consistently dull" rat. The consistently dull rat doesn't do particularly well in any of the available environments (see figure 3.3). What will happen to the heritability of maze-running ability if we add this hypothetical rat into our population? It will increase. Conversely, if we had started with such a rat in our experiment, and we removed it from the population, heritability would decrease. We might call these changes in the genotypic *range* of the population. Obviously, changes in the genotypic range are closely related to changes in the genotypic *frequency.* Indeed, changes in the range can be thought of as just

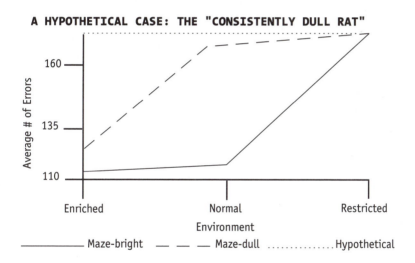

Data for Figure 3.3

Average number of errors for three types of rats (one of which is hypothetical) in three types of environments:

Environment/Rat Type	Enriched	Normal	Restricted
Maze-bright	111.2	117	169.7
Maze-dull	119.7	164	169.5
Hypothetical	169	169	169

Figure 3.3: The addition of a hypothetical "consistently dull" rat to the population.

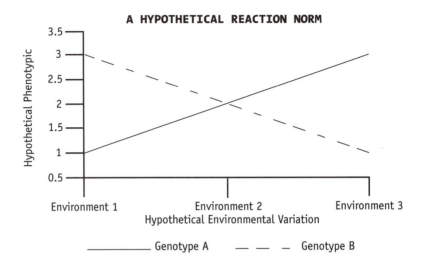

Data for Figure 3.4

Hypothetical phenotype scores for two hypothetical genotypes in three hypothetical environments:

Environment/Genotype	Environment 1	Environment 2	Environment 3
Genotype A	1	2	3
Genotype B	3	2	1

Figure 3.4: A hypothetical reaction norm.

---

rather special cases of changes in frequency. So, changes where the frequency goes to zero are reductions in the range, and changes where the frequency increases upward from zero are increases in the range. However, changes in the range *are* a special case, and thinking of them as distinct is worthwhile.

Would knowing that the heritability of a trait was zero tell us anything of interest? Would it, for example, imply that there were no genetic differences in the population that were relevant to the trait? Again, the answer is no. Consider figure 3.4 (adapted from Lewontin 1974). Here, the heritability of the trait across the environments in question is zero (and so is the environmentality). Neither genotype does better overall, nor is any particular environment better overall. It is clear, however, that there is an important difference in how the genotypes respond to the environments. Indeed, if the distribution of the organisms into environments was shifted so that most found themselves to the right, suddenly the heritability of the trait in question would be large. Indeed, it we paid attention to only *part* of the environmental range, we would find significant heritability.

It is occasionally suggested that while knowing the heritability of a trait doesn't give any "final" answers, it is a good "first step" toward understanding the effects of genes and the environment within a particular population. Plomin et al. write that while heritability alone cannot be taken to be a guide to what "could be" it is "important to begin with what is: the genetic and environmental sources of variance in existing populations" (1997, 84). When researchers are quoted to the effect that high heritability estimates are "suggestive" (Goldman, quoted in Kitcher 1999, n. 11), they seem to be motioning in the same direction. However, it is dubious that even such apparently cautious views as those can be adequately defended. If what you want to do is explain the causal source of the current variation, or predict what kinds of changes, in, say, the distributions of environments or the population will have what kinds of effects, you *need* to know the reaction norms for the traits in questions; heritability estimates alone, no matter how accurate, will never suffice. By now it should be clear that very different reaction norms can have, based on local features of the population, the exact same heritability. Another way of putting the point is that radically different underlying mechanisms, in terms of the developmental biology, say, can lie behind a given quantitative finding, such as an estimate of heritability. Without additional information, there is no way of telling even what *kind* of mechanism is behind the sort of statistical result heritability estimates involve (see Pigliucci and Schlichting 1997; Pigliucci 1996; Schlichting and Pigliucci 1998; Bailey 1997).

Even if you know the heritability of trait, and even if that heritability is quite high, if you don't know the norm of reaction for the trait in question and the environments and organisms in question, it is *in principle* impossible to predict what kinds of effects various possible changes in the population will have on the trait in question. Again, in a population of Cooper and Zubek's maze-bright and maze-dull rats, if most of them were raised in the "normal" environment, heritability would be very high indeed. Does this mean that changes in the environments the rats were raised in would have minimal effects on eliminating differences between the strains? Not at all—when raised in *either* a "restricted" or an "enriched" environment, all the statistically significant variations between the strains of rats vanish. As we saw above, Jung claimed that the high heritability of obesity made it an "actual disease" (1997). Is this plausible? Does a high heritability mean that the trait in question is in some way a "real" trait?

Not, I think we would be inclined to say, if you are measuring the allometric response of one trait that varies *because* some other trait is responding to the environment in question (say),[15] or is under relatively direct genetic influence (say), but has no particular biological significance itself (see for example Gould and Lewontin 1978; Pigliucci et al. 1996; Schlichting and Pigliucci 1998). As for being able to say something coherent about causation given nothing but the heritability of a trait, it seems clear that extreme caution is warranted. To say that a high heritability implies that the variation in a trait is *caused* mostly by the genetic variation should strike us as awkward. Without additional information no predictions can be made on the basis of this causal claim, it seems inadequate for explaining the variations of interest, and the underlying causal structure remains entirely opaque.

Conclusion
Heritability is difficult to calculate in human populations. Because of its strictly local nature, it is at best of very limited use, and likely of no use in explaining differences in traits that matter to us in human populations or for predicting how such traits will respond to changes in the environment. These limitations, as will become clear, in turn make heritability almost useless for formulating any policy decisions that surround these traits. It is indeed somewhat unclear what knowing the heritability of a trait in a particular population of people would tell us; that is, it is unclear what interpretation should be given the number.

However, heritability estimates are still widely cited, and suggestions about their possible use are still common. One reason for this can be seen in surveys of what we know about the genetics of various complex human traits: often all that is known about the relationship of genetics to some trait is the heritability of that trait (see for example Plomin et al. 1990, 1997; Plomin 1990; Hamer and Copeland 1998; Loehlin 1992). If heritability estimates were to be disregarded (again, as many biologists feel they should be), the field of human genetics research (and especially human behavior genetics) would be left with far less "data" than it currently has.

In the next chapters, as some human traits of popular interest are discussed, some specific uses of heritability estimates will be critiqued, in part using the framework developed here.

"Finding Genes": Linkage and Molecular Genetics

Much of the current excitement in the popular press surrounding human genetics research comes from "finding the gene" for some trait, or, in more cautious moments, "finding *a* gene" for some trait. Over the past decade, increasingly large numbers of claims have been made for the discovery of the genes associated with "high intelligence," "depression," "obesity," "violence," "risk-seeking behavior," and a range of other complex traits in humans, as well as relatively simpler diseases such as Alzheimer's disease, various early-onset forms of breast cancer, and the like. In this section, I will briefly outline what the basic approach to "finding genes" in humans associated with various traits is, and discuss some of the limitations that these approaches have.

Very crudely put, the basic technique for "discovering" genes associated with a given trait in humans is to compare the genomes of individuals with and without the trait of interest. If those with the trait of interest share a segment of their genome more often than those without it, this is taken to be evidence that somewhere in the area of interest is a gene that influences the trait in question. Further analysis can then "home in" on the gene in question, which can then be sequenced. This can provide information about what protein the gene in question produces, which, it is thought, can yield some insights into the biochemical basis of the trait.[16]

While it is becoming relatively common to find and sequence genes associated with radically abnormal conditions,[17] finding genes associated with variations in the "normal" part of the spectrum of behavioral or other phenotypic traits in humans has proven more difficult.[18] Indeed, even the discovery of genes associated with mental diseases such as depression and schizophrenia has proven to be very tricky, and those discoveries that have been announced have often proven to be difficult to replicate (see Horgan 1993 for a general survey; for a survey of recent claims surrounding molecular findings in bipolar affective disorders, see Baron 1997). In any case, what "finding genes" in any of these cases actually teaches you is a bit of an open question.

For conditions that are part of the spectrum of "normal" traits, where a gene has been located that is thought to influence the trait in question but has not been sequenced, extreme caution in interpreting the results is advisable. Indeed, even if the gene has been sequenced, unless there is a firm understanding of the biochemical and especially the developmental pathways the gene is involved in, it is difficult to determine what we have learned in "discovering" the gene. Again, this is because particular forms of the gene in question may have certain kinds of effects under some developmental conditions, but not in others. So, for example, a particular form of a gene might be associated with a particular deviation from the mean value for a given trait in some developmental environments but not in others. Further, interactions with other genes may also change the way a particular form of a gene is related to a particular trait, so that a gene may have a particular effect only if other particular genes are present (see Pigliucci and Schlichting 1997 for a summary and discussion of some of these problems). Both these difficulties are focused on the *context dependence* of the effects that genes have; in the first case, it was the environmental context, and in the second case, it was a broader genetic context. As many biologists now accept that these forms of context dependence are the rule rather than the exception (see Pigliucci and Schlichting 1997; Schlichting and Pigliucci 1998; and references therein), it is important that the limitations they impose be taken seriously.

As we do not yet have a firm understanding of all, or even most, of the developmental pathways involved in any complex human trait, these cautions should be taken very seriously indeed. It is likely that most human traits of interest are the result of complex interactions between many clusters of genes and many environmental variables. Schlichting and Pigliucci note that even the usual way of conceiving of these traits as being "polygenic" is "too narrow" because the traits in questions may not be "directly" controlled by genes at all. Rather, they may be "the result of complex epigenetic interactions and emergent outcomes of developmental systems, only remotely connected with the DNA level" (1998, 337). Does this mean that we shouldn't expect to find genetic influences on these traits if we look for them? Not at all. Since the same complex characteristics "are controlled to some extent by genes," it is possible to find "localized" gene actions if one is looking for them (Schlichting and Pigliucci 1998, 337). It does mean, I think, that we ought not to take those "influences" we do find too seriously, if what we are attempting to do with them involves in any way making predictions about or explaining variations in those complex traits we care about. If our goal is merely a methodological one of using gene sequencing as an entry point into an attempt to, say, "unravel the neurochemistry" of some disorder by using the "molecular details" as a "thread that will lead [researchers] into the" complexities of brain chemistry and reactions (as Kitcher would have it—see Kitcher 1999, 23), these problems are not so pressing. However, insofar as our goals are related to social policy decisions or causal explanations, "finding a gene" can barely be considered a first step toward those goals, and will, again, generally be irrelevant unless many more steps are taken.

The problem in which genes may have certain kinds of influences on the phenotype of an organism in certain developmental environments and not others is closely related to a more general observation. *Reaction norms* (see above, and for an example see figure 3.1) are a graphical representation of the way that particular forms of genes can interact with a developmental environment to produce different kinds of phenotypes. Organisms can and often do display "plastic" phenotypes (traits that vary according to the environments, developmental and otherwise, that they are expressed in); indeed, the evolution of "plasticity" is now a hot topic in developmental and evolutionary biology (see Schlichting and Pigliucci 1998). If, as seems prima facie likely, many of the genes for the phenotypic traits of interest to us in human genetics (intelligence, temperament, sexuality, etc.) are involved in any of the various sorts of plasticity known to exist, caution about what claims a given finding will support is warranted. Again, while a gene may be associated with a particular

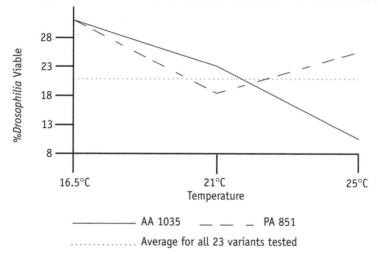

DROSOPHILA VIABILITY: TWO VARIANTS COMPARED TO THE AVERAGE

——————— AA 1035   — —   — PA 851

.... Average for all 23 variants tested

Data for Figure 3.5

Percent of *Drosophila* viable at three different temperatures for two different genotypes and the average of 23 tested genotypes:

Temperature/Genotype	16.5°C	21°C	25.5°C
AA 1035	30.29	23.23	10.23
PA 851	30.54	18.97	26.35
Average for all 23 variants tested	20.86	20.5	18.9

Figure 3.5: The percentage of Drosophila *viable at given temperatures. Notice that both variants are superior to average in some environments but inferior in others.*

variation on a trait in one environment, it may not be associated with it in another, or indeed may be associated with some quite different variation on that trait.

For example, an allele (a form of a gene) that is associated with higher than average larval viability in *Drosophila* in one environment can be associated with *lower* than average larval viability in a different one (see figure 3.5; the data for this example comes from Dobzhansky and Spassky 1944, reprinted in Lewontin et al., eds., 1981). Indeed, at least in the chromosomal variants of *Drosophila* that Dobzhansky tested, "not a single chromosome gave viability records superior to normal at all the temperatures" (377). A search for genes associated with, say, high viability, undertaken in the *Drosophila* that Dobzhansky studied, would, if done at a particular temperature, yield a result that held *only* for that temperature—in other temperatures the gene would *not* necessarily be associated with high viability anymore.

It should be noted that the same could be said of *environments* as well. Any claim for finding a particular environment that was better for viability in the *Drosophila* and temperatures that Dobzhansky studied would be equally unfounded. Some variants do best at low temperatures, some at the middle temperature tested, and others at higher temperatures (see figure 3.6). Indeed, notice that PA 851 does better at the two extreme environments tested and worse at the middle one! Which temperature is "best" for *Drosophila* viability depends on which genetic variant of *Drosophila* one is dealing with. There is no more reason to think there are universally best environments than that there are universally best genes. This quite general point is too often overlooked in the endless "nature versus nurture" debates. It will become an important issue in the discussions of particular research projects that follow, especially those related to temperament and mood-affective disorders and those related to intelligence and IQ test scores.

Of course, there are genes that are *terrible* in almost all environments, and environments that are terrible to almost all relevant genotypes. In the case of the *Drosophila* tested by Dobzhansky, a few strains did terribly in all the temperatures tested; two of these strains, AA 1005 and AA 1212, are shown, with the average for comparison, in figure 3.7. And while no temperature tested was worse for every kind of *Drosophila*, it doesn't take much imagination to realize that some would have been—for example, all those above 100°C or well below freezing! In humans, we know that many genetic diseases are caused by single-gene disorders and have severe effects in every known environment (see Plomin et al. 1990, 59ff., 83ff., 127ff.). And we know that some environments are terrible for people to

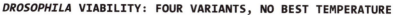

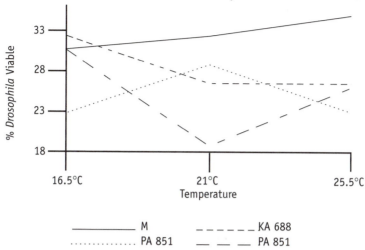

Data for Figure 3.6

Percent of *Drosophila* viable at three different temperatures for four different genotypes:

Temperature/Genotype	16.5°C	21°C	25.5°C
M	30.6	31.89	34.14
KA 688	32.2	26.83	26.85
AA 1052	23.31	28.23	23.52
PA 851	30.54	18.97	26.35

Figure 3.6: The percentage of Drosophila *viable at three temperatures for four different variants. Note that no temperature is better for every kind of Drosophila.*

develop in, such as those environments where they are constantly exposed to large quantities of lead dust or get very little attention from other humans. But the basic point—that *in general* knowing the genotype or knowing the environment alone is not enough to predict relative success without knowing how they *interact*—holds for many of the cases that have been explored, especially those on the "normal" part of the spectrum.

Epistatic effects, the interactions of genes with other genes, are now recognized as "pervasive" (Pigliucci and Schlichting 1997, 150) and of enormous importance to understanding the evolution and development

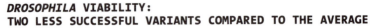

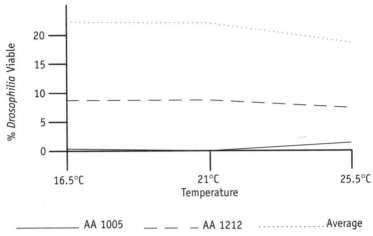

DROSOPHILA VIABILITY:
TWO LESS SUCCESSFUL VARIANTS COMPARED TO THE AVERAGE

AA 1005 — — — AA 1212 ·············· Average

Data for Figure 3.7

Percent of *Drosophila* viable at three different temperatures for two different genotypes and the average of 23 tested varieties:

Temperature/Genotype	16.5°C	21°C	25.5°C
AA 1005	0.29	0.069	1.21
AA 1212	8.63	8.54	7.03
Average	20.86	20.5	18

Figure 3.7: The reaction norms for two strains of Drosophila *that were much less successful than average at all temperatures tested. Notice that even so, one strain does better at the higher temperatures, the other does better at the lower temperatures.*

of organisms (see Schlichting and Pigliucci 1998, esp. ch. 9).[19] In one form of epistatic effect, genes that have a given effect in some genetic contexts will not have that effect in others. Again, recognition of the pervasiveness of epistatic effects recommends caution in the interpretation of studies that claim to have found a gene associated with some trait where the biochemical developmental pathways and other details have not been properly elucidated. A gene that has a positive influence on some trait in some genetic contexts may well lack that effect in other genetic contexts;

indeed, genes with a positive influence on a trait in one genetic context may, in a different genetic context, even have a negative influence on the trait (see Pigliucci and Schlichting 1997; Schlichting and Pigliucci 1998; Altenberg and Wagner 1996; and citations therein for an examination of how such effects can evolve and be maintained). The assumption that a gene that has a positive effect in one genetic context will have a positive effect in every genetic context turns out to be false. Nevertheless, this assumption—that genes that interact with each other in these cases will do so in an additive way—is often made. For traits that vary quantitatively, the assumption of additivity is largely necessary for the search for "quantitative trait loci" (multiple genes that each influence the trait in question somewhat) to make sense. Without the assumption of additivity, finding an association between one form of the gene in question and one kind of variation in the trait would not permit claims about the influence that form of the gene had "in general" on the trait (positive, negative, or neutral). Indeed, the question might not even make sense.

The caution recommended in interpreting the results of studies that claim to find a gene associated with a condition but do little to elucidate a plausible developmental pathway from the gene to the trait in question, then, is that these results are by necessity restricted. So, for example, a gene found to be "associated" with "high IQ" in one context—that is, in either one set of environments or in one kind of genetic environment—may not be associated with "high IQ" in other environments, or even in all the environments available.[20] Notice, for example, that in figure 3.6 one of the variants does better than average overall, but worse than average in one of the three available environments.

As noted above, so far at least the vast majority of work that has begun to elucidate any of the complex biochemical and developmental pathways from genes to phenotypes in humans has been done on relatively simple genetic diseases. Until such work is done on traits where variations within the "normal" range are of interest to us, the promise that someday genetics research will be in a position to elucidate such causal pathways must remain just that: a promise. Given that, claims about *understanding* the genetics behind a condition, or claims about what "discovering a gene" associated with some conditions *means*, say, for policy decisions, should be greeted with skepticism. Indeed, many biologists would now argue that until we know not only about what is going on at the molecular level, and understand how this fits into not only the organism's development but also the overall evolutionary context of the organism, including ecological contexts and the like, we shouldn't claim to understand the genetics behind the trait in question, or claim to be able to predict how the trait in

MONTROSE LIBRARY DISTRICT
320 So. 2nd St.
Montrose, CO 81401

question will respond to various sorts of possible changes (Pigliucci, personal communication 1998; see also Bailey 1997, 129–30, on the "fallacy of salvation in technology").

"Evolutionary Reasoning" and the Evolution of (Phenotypic) Variation

Until relatively recently, most of the work that went on in fitting complex human traits (behaviors and otherwise) into an evolutionary framework was focused on explaining features that were thought to be *universal* to humans (see Plomin et al. 1997, 243). These approaches, made famous by Wilson's 1975 book *Sociobiology: The New Synthesis*, attempted to explain human behaviors and other complex traits on the basis of their value to the evolutionary fitness of the organism in question. The promise of this project was premised on the idea of inclusive fitness; that is, the extent to which the trait may have helped not only the reproductive success of the individual displaying it but related individuals as well, who would be more likely to possess copies of the same genes and pass them on than the population at large (see Dawkins's *The Selfish Gene*, 1976). Whatever the merits of and problems with these conceptual strategies—and many people argue that the problems, even with recent articulations, far outweigh the merits[21]—they are of little interest in thinking about human differences.[22] What is of interest to us here are those research programs that, rather than trying to discern and explain universals in human behavior by reference to some proposed evolutionary story, attempt to use evolutionary stories to explain the *variations* that exist in complex human traits.

There are any number of conceptions how this sort of project could be developed, and what in fact it means. Some authors write as if what we should expect are relatively stable equilibrium states of organisms (humans) engaged in different strategies (see for example Hamer and Copeland 1998, 48–49). Others write as if the genetic influence is not on the variation that exists between individuals, but rather on the ability of individuals themselves to adopt different strategies;[23] this is another way of expressing the claim that we should expect that the traits in question are "plastic" with respect to the environments encountered. Generally, the arguments that link up to the molecular approaches as well as quantitative approaches, such as studies estimating heritability, are of the former sort; that is, they hypothesize that the variation that exists is related (directly) to the genetic variation in the population, and not to the plasticity of the trait. Both these approaches are discussed in some detail below.

Another kind of argument that is sometimes seen is that the traits in question are not important enough from an evolutionary standpoint to have been selected for or against, or that the evolution of such traits is "constrained" by their links with other traits (epigenetic effects and genetic covariances). On this argument, variation is maintained not actively but because there was no force acting strongly enough to get rid of it (see for example Loehlin 1992, 123). The point of these arguments is not to show that variation must exist and be genetically influenced, but rather that there is no reason why it could not be. This approach is not popular among most writers involved in thinking about the possible relationship of genetic variation to the variation within complex human traits, possibly because it often makes those traits out to seem less important than the writers would like to think. While it is very hard to show that variation in some complex human trait could not be related to evolutionarily neutral genetic variation, it is also, for somewhat obvious reasons, hard to show that variation in some trait *is* related to evolutionarily neutral genetic variation. For that reason, this approach will not be discussed in as much detail, and the (few) specific uses made of it in discussions of the specific cases brought out later in this work will be treated individually.

The Evolution of Variation: Individuals with Different Traits
The basic idea behind arguments that purport to show that it is reasonable to expect that the variations between people with respect to some trait would be maintained if the trait were under some form of genetic control is to show that there is an evolutionarily stable equilibrium state where the population is "mixed"; that is, where different members have different versions of the trait. The traditional way to think through these examples is to find some model where in some population in which everyone has a given version of some trait, someone with an alternate version of that trait would do "better"; that is, would have greater reproductive success. This would drive the proportion of people with the alternate form up. In cases where stable equilibriums form, once a certain number of people have the alternate form of the trait, increases in the proportion will actually be selected against. The claim that some "evolutionarily stable strategies" involve stable polymorphisms is just the claim that some evolutionarily stable states are equilibriums with various different "strategies" being played simultaneously. The existence of such situations has been well established both theoretically and, to a somewhat lesser extent, empirically (see for example Shaw 1958).

As applied to complex human traits, it is difficult if not impossible to imagine cases where the contention that variations have been maintained in this manner could be adequately tested. However, various authors have suggested evolutionarily stable polymorphisms as a possible explanation for the continued existence of variation. So Hamer and Copeland, for example, hypothesize that the variation that exists in human "novelty seeking" may have been maintained in this manner. They start by arguing that the variation that exists is probably in some significant part due to genetic variation. They claim that this follows from quantitative research —namely an estimated heritability for novelty seeking of about 40 percent—as well as from molecular research—namely their having "found" a gene that is correlated with risk-seeking behavior, albeit one that "accounted" for a very small proportion of the differences (Hamer and Copeland 1998, 46). Of course, one must keep in mind the limitations, of the sorts discussed above, on what quantitative studies and molecular "finding the gene" studies can show. In any event, Hamer and Copeland then wonder how this variation could have been maintained. They note that within a given population, both risk seekers and risk avoiders (and indeed, "moderates') can be successful. For example, risk seekers might sometimes reap huge rewards by taking risks, and risk avoiders might prevent disaster by being very cautious. In the right circumstance, each strategy could prove advantageous in terms of reproductive success. At different times, and in different local environments, both types of people, Hamer and Copeland argue, will do well. It is further implied that in a population of all risk seekers, a cautious person would likely do better than average; in a population of all cautious people, a risk seeker might well do better. The "equilibrium point" will be somewhere between the extremes. Different environments, they note, might foster different percentages, but the basic idea would be the same (47–49).[24]

Again, it is hard to see how positive evidence *for* the maintenance of such polymorphisms involving complex human traits in natural human populations could be found. As was noted above, simply finding a gene (or set of genes) where differences at the genetic level are correlated with differences in the traits involved isn't enough to justify the claim that these genes are, in any strong sense, *for* the particular versions of the trait. The problems, again, are that (a) an organism with a given genotype may have a very different phenotype for the trait concerned if the environment is different (phenotypic plasticity); (b) different genes may respond differently to the environment;—that is, different genes may have different reaction norms; and (c) the relationship between the trait in question and gene in question may be artifact of the complex relationship the gene has with other "suites" of traits, a problem related to the complexities posed by epigenetic effects and genetic covariances. So without knowing the complex relationship between the context of the gene and the resulting phenotype—without, in other words, knowing about the epigenetic effects and the norms of reaction for the genes in question—guesses about the evolutionary significance of the variation found must remain just that—guesses.

However, as long as the arguments are phrased as attempts to explain merely how it is *possible* that variations in complex traits could have been actively maintained in an evolutionary context, these problems are not so biting. But it would be generally agreed, I think, that it is an error to argue from the theoretical possibility of such evolutionarily stable polymorphisms to the conclusion that the variations we actually find are the result of such polymorphisms—possibility is *not* the same thing as actuality. So while it is hard to argue with such explanations being offered to account for the possibility of variation, attempts to explain actual variation by reference to such explanations should probably be regarded with some skepticism. While Hamer and Copeland are relatively careful to not move beyond the claim that such polymorphisms are a possibility, their claim that it is "probably more important" that the different evolutionary strategies (high versus low thrill seeking) might be associated with different sexual strategies does seem to imply that an explanation of actual variation in the population is being proffered, and not just a purely hypothetical case.[25] In any event, one should certainly resist the temptation to interpret claims that follow from these sorts of stories in any but the most cautious way.

The Evolution of Plasticity
Rather than searching for differences in traits associated with differences in genes, one could approach the question of trying to untangle the causes of variations in complex human traits by attempting to figure out how the development of those traits is influenced by the interaction of particular genes with the environmental and genetic contexts in which they appear. In some cases, complex human traits might respond to differences in the environments (developmental or otherwise) encountered, and it would be interesting and valuable to know something about both how and why they varied. The variations of this sort that would be of note to someone interested in thinking about the way that genetic differences can be associated with phenotypic differences would be those variations *in the response* of the genes to environmental variations; that is, explorations of genes associated with phenotypic plasticity.

By far the most satisfactory explorations of the evolution of phenotypic plasticity in humans would be research following the sort that is beginning to yield results in, for example, some species of plants and some other model organisms (see for example Pigliucci 1999; Pigliucci et al. 1999a; Schmitt et al. 1999, and references therein). Here, the mechanisms by which phenotypic plasticity—the ability of organisms to change, often in complex ways, in response to different environments—are studied in relation to the evolutionary history and ecology of the organisms in question. An explanation of the variation in complex human traits that made use of the range of techniques brought out by authors interested in relatively simple traits in plants would be welcome indeed. A study of this sort would finally be a way of really exploring the relationship between the genetic and the environmental influences on the traits in question. In some cases, for some traits, it might of course turn out that there is not much plasticity at all; in others, there might be quite a lot. Unfortunately, there is no data on how the development of any complex human traits respond to different environments, nor is there likely to be any in the foreseeable future.

Sadly, the basic requirements for generating any reaction norms— that one have access to organisms with relevantly similar genotypes, and that one be able to raise them in environments that vary according to the environmental variables whose interaction with the genotype in question one wishes to study—make such studies impossible on humans (see for example Lewontin 1974). Indeed, even in plants, sometimes interpreting the data that is generated when norms of reaction are successfully developed for relatively simple traits can prove to be tricky (see Pigliucci et al. 1999b). This is further cause for pessimism about the chances that convincing reaction norms for the interaction of any genes and any complex human traits for any interesting environments will be imminently forthcoming.

Conclusion: Explaining Variation in Complex Human Traits

In the coming chapters, we will be looking at specific examples of complex human traits where it has been claimed that (a) research has shown us something interesting about the relationship between genetic variation in the population and variation in the trait of interest, and (b) this interesting thing about the relationship has some implications for how we should think about the trait, such as social or public policy implications, or implications for moral judgments. The argument I want to make in these cases is similarly twofold. First, I will argue that the "interesting thing" that the research has shown is of much more limited value (and interest) than most accounts of it would make it appear. This is especially true of those that occur in the popular press, but also holds for those accounts that appear in reputable peer-reviewed journals. Second, I will argue that the research that has been undertaken and reported *so far* does not support the claimed implications it was supposed to have.

Recent research and claims in the popular press have tended to focus on the genetic as the primary source for variation, and so, by default, my arguments will often stress that other explanations involving complex gene-environment interactions (for example) or environmental variations are not excluded by the data we have now. But I will *not* be arguing that it *is* the environment that "causes" the variation, or even that it is actually complex interactions between genes and their contexts. For many of the traits of interest to us, I would argue, there is no better evidence for *those* claims now, nor any better way of gathering evidence for claims like those, than for the hypotheses centered on genetic causes and explanations that I will be arguing against. But in another circumstance, should environmental influences be taken to be all powerful, and people set out in search of the "best" environment, the same arguments could obviously be applied against those sorts of claims as well. Now, however, most of the excitement is surrounding genes and genetic explanations, and so that is where the arguments will be focused.

CHAPTER 4

IQ AND SOCIAL POLICY

The Old and the New

In this chapter I consider the claims that have been made about the relationship between genes and intelligence in light of the limitations on what human genetic research can show that were pointed out in the last chapters. In the case of studies of heritability, the last chapters provided some general reasons to be suspicious about the usefulness of the concept of broad-sense heritability in thinking about those variations in significant human behaviors and traits. Because of the conceptual limitations to heritability, it was argued that heritability estimates were neither useful for making predictions about changing variations in traits nor for explaining those variations that currently exist in naturally occurring populations without knowing far more about how the purported genes involved interacted with the environment (and other aspects of their contexts). It was further argued that arriving at convincing estimates of the heritability of complex traits in human populations was at best difficult. However, it was noted that none of these problems, well-known as they are, have stopped people from embarking on research designed to generate such estimates, from publishing such estimates, or from using such estimates in arguments about social policy.

Perhaps the best known case is the use of estimates of the heritability of performance on IQ tests.[1] While estimating the heritability of a trait like performance on IQ tests in humans is difficult, if not impossible (see chapter 3), this hasn't prevented people from trying, nor from publishing their results. Indeed, the numbers for the heritability of IQ scores that emerge from the projects that attempt to do so have become generally accepted in the popular press and in the discussions of the issues that surround these numbers. So, for example, following the results of Bouchard's so-called Minnesota Twin Study, heritability estimates of about .7, or 70 percent, are often cited (Bouchard, see various publications 1990ff.). However accurate or inaccurate this number is, it is of course more important that the interpretations often given to the heritability of performance on IQ tests in humans are implausible at best.

Recently, some researchers who had been involved with heritability studies on performance on IQ tests have turned their attention to molecular-genetic approaches, attempting to find genes associated with variations in "intelligence" as measured by IQ and other standardized tests. Some researchers and popular authors have taken the reported successes at finding genes so associated as evidence that the heritability estimates, as well as the claims made about the implications of high heritability, are at least on the right track (for a summary of some of these arguments and the studies that they are based on, see Daniels et al. 1996).

This chapter will primarily be concerned with the use of heritability estimates and the findings of molecular genetics research to make claims about the inevitability or naturalness of social ranking in the United States. This is an especially troubling argument when it is applied to those differences in socioeconomic status (SES) and access to power resources that fall along so-called ethnic (or racial) differences within the different populations in the United States. This sort of interpretation, it will be argued, is entirely insupportable by both the data available, and, more importantly, by the very conceptual apparatus used in estimating the heritability of performance on IQ tests or in finding genes associated with variations in performance on various tests meant to measure intelligence.

Another interpretation often made of the claimed high heritability of performance on IQ tests and the recent molecular genetics findings is not that this somehow explains or justifies current or possible distributions of power and wealth within society, but rather that it points toward certain policies in education and away from others. Usually the argument goes something like this: Intelligence is largely genetic, so education won't really help people who are doing poorly, so education dollars are more or less wasted on people who aren't that smart, and, although this is rarely made explicit, would be better spent on children who already are smart (this argument is made most famously in Jensen 1969, but Jensen 1982 makes it even more explicit, and Murray and Herrnstein 1994 often imply much the same thing).

In bringing out the sorts of errors that are made in these arguments, I will start in what might seem an unlikely place—I will return to Cooper and Zubek's study of maze-running ability in rats, which was discussed in the previous chapter. This study, if you will recall, was of some interest in thinking about heritability in part because it so clearly demonstrated why arguments from a high heritability of some trait in some population in a given distribution of environments to its inevitability in other environments are deeply mistaken. After looking at this case again, some of the old arguments about so-called ethnic differences and differences in IQ scores will be reviewed, along with the old counterarguments. If the arguments that currently get attention were startlingly different then the old ones, this would be a waste of time, but, far from startlingly different, the new versions of these arguments are very nearly the same. In going through the newer versions of these arguments, I will try to draw attention to the way that the conceptual limitations of the techniques they rely on make their conclusions insupportable. Next, I will argue that even the recent and relatively less contentious claims that move from recent research results in human genetics, whether quantitative or more molecularly minded, to conclusions about the at best small possible effects of education, or environmental changes, or the like, are flawed for much the same reasons. In going through them, and some of the contemporary attacks on these arguments, I hope it becomes clear that these kinds of interpretations, even when they don't sound completely wrongheaded, are utterly insupportable without the addition of huge numbers of unargued for, and utterly insupportable, assumptions.

Rats in a Maze: Learning Ability and Environmental Variation

To briefly review what was said about Cooper and Zubek's work in the last chapter, the experiment involved rats bred to run mazes with relatively few errors ("maze-bright") or with relatively many errors ("maze-dull"). In the "normal" environment (the one in which selection took place) the average number of errors made by the two strains of rats were very different; in both the "enriched" and "impoverished" environments, however, the two strains of rats performed roughly equally. As we saw in the last chapter, in the normal environment, the heritability of maze-running ability would be quite high, but if the populations were concentrated on just the two modified environments, the heritability of maze-running ability would of course have been very low or nonexistent (see figure 3.1 and box 3.2). Consider again the distribution of the population into the possible environments. As we saw in the last chapter, a population in which most of the rats were in either the enriched or the restricted environments would have a very low heritability for maze-running ability; one in which most of the rats were in the normal environment would have a high heritability for maze-running ability.

Interestingly, a distressingly common reaction to the results of this study is to claim that the researchers actually failed to breed for maze-running ability at all, and instead bred for something else that had the *effect* of influencing maze-running ability in that one environment. Henderson, apparently, claimed that further research on the strains hinted that it is motivation and curiosity that were the real issues in the strains Cooper and Zubek had bred. Further, he claimed that in other strains, with which he worked, there was a "real" difference in learning ability "per se" and that in those strains environment and rearing made much less difference (Henderson 1972; see Plomin et al. 1990, 270ff. and Plomin et al. 1997, 131ff. for a discussion of these experiments.)

But this response misses the point entirely. The strains that Cooper and Zubek worked with were selected for maze-running ability; in the case of the maze-bright rats, they were selected to be good at maze-running, and in the case of maze-dull rats they were selected to be bad at maze-running. The claim that in the environment where selection took place, maze-running ability was mediated by motivation and curiosity, and that this is what was "really" selected for in the rats, could only make sense if traits could exist independently of environments (more on this issue in chapter 10). But there can be no maze-running ability without an environment, and in the environment of selection, the rats were clearly selected to be maze-bright or maze-dull rats in as powerful a way as selection can work. The "evolutionary pressure" was extraordinarily high, to use the metaphor. The unpredictability of what will happen to traits selected for in one environment when they are placed in another one is the very point, not a problem with the test.[2]

But why reject the significance of Henderson's results? After all, it might be claimed, he found a way to get rats that are *really* maze-bright and maze-dull, that *really* differ in their learning ability "per se." Henderson attempted to isolate "learning ability" from other traits by creating situations in which "motivation" was uniformly high and curiosity irrelevant— tasks such as escaping from electric shocks or water. That there were major strain differences and that these differences didn't respond to early environmental effects he took as evidence that "learning ability" didn't show rearing effects or genotype-environment interaction (Plomin 1990, 270). However, it is unclear why one would think of learning ability in environments in which motivation and curiosity are irrelevant as in any way more constitutive of learning ability "per se" than those in which those traits are key. That is, a conception of learning ability that makes it out to be deeply wrapped up in curiosity and motivation may strike us as at least as central a conception of learning ability as one that doesn't. What *counts* as learning ability, what is a part of learning ability, and what is something separable from it that merely *looks* like a part of learning ability is at the very least not a trivial issue.

We might be suspicious of Henderson's results on other grounds as well. His studies on learning in rats were done using several different strains of much more heavily inbred lines of rats than those that Cooper and Zubek used. Henderson's rats were not bred specifically for any special learning task, but instead simply to be genetically homogeneous. As it turns out, some commercial rat strains do worse than others on standard learning tests, pretty much across the board. And some commercial rat strains show little environmental or rearing effects in many of the tests commonly performed. But in all these cases, the rats in the trials were created by massive inbreeding, which often results in "inbreeding depression"—the "general malaise of inbred individuals caused by the increase in homozygosity" (Plomin et al. 1990, 195; see also 285). Some rat strains are just hopelessly bogged down by their total homozygosity; others have fewer problems. Various different strains of homozygotic rats have different levels and sorts of problems, depending on how deleterious is the given form of homozygosity they happened to have latched on to. Whether or not Henderson's rats suffered any of these sorts of problems, the point here is that the rats in question weren't *normal* (relevantly similar to wild) rats at all. One can legitimately question whether results one gets from using rats that genetically have been badly abused should be expanded to other situations.

For the most part, though, even among those massively inbred, hopelessly bogged-down strains, there is no regularity to their performance in various tasks. Except for the most hopelessly listless and stupid, it turns out that strains that learn faster on some tasks will often learn slower on others, with little in the way of regularity. Indeed, what amount to the "best" conditions for learning are different for different strains and for different given tasks. For example, some strains learn better (faster) if the trials are spread out, and others if the trials are massed (Plomin et al. 1990, 268). The environment of learning obviously makes a difference to these animals, and strains that are faster in one learning situation will often turn out to be slower in another.

A more interesting problem with Cooper and Zubek's experiment on learning ability in rats is that it is somewhat obvious that environments cannot be easily ranked in a well-ordered continuous way from "restricted" to "enriched"—either for rats in laboratory cages, or indeed more generally. In the case of Cooper and Zubek's experiment, the problem was avoided by having environments that were obviously very far apart in terms of available levels of stimulation. These included environments of truly massive deprivation. However, it is unclear what implications environments so different from each other have for thinking about more subtle, and ordinary, differences in environments. And this is actually a serious problem in thinking about the relationship between IQ scores and environments more generally. The continual rise of IQ scores in the developed world over the past several decades (the so-called Flynn effect) is sometimes attributed to "better" environments (see Block 1995, 124). This is despite the fact that there is very little data available on what sorts of environments are better and worse for performance on IQ tests or how they have the effects they do, *except* for the information we have on environments that are *awful* for performance on IQ tests—for example, environments that are nutritionally massively deprived, seriously toxic, and so on (see Block 1995, 118–19). How the changing environment over the past decades has had a beneficial effect on performance on IQ tests remains unclear, as does what forms of intervention would be effective in, for example, boosting the effect or even ensuring its continuation.

However, the basic intention here was to point out how important the environment could be to estimates of heritability, and to point out how changes in the environment could make apparently large differences that can be attributed to genetic differences simply *vanish*. This result doesn't require much subtlety; the problem with ranking environments is a problem of being able to *quantify* these differences and make predictions about what will happen when various kinds of small changes are made. But as we shall see, once it becomes clear that the interpretations of the heritability of performance on IQ tests are completely irrelevant from the standpoint of predicting what the effects that, for example, changes in educational policies could be expected to have in society at large, the temptation to attempt these kinds of quantitative analyses will, I hope, have been purged.

Race and IQ

Arguments to the effect that differences in the economic status or social success between various ethic or racial groups could be best accounted for by intrinsic differences among the members of the groups, especially differences between the average levels of "intelligence," have a very long history. Kevles, in his brilliant 1985 book *In the Name of Eugenics*, traces the last hundred years or so of such "scientific" arguments. For roughly the last thirty years, arguments of this sort have been based on the (supposed) high heritability of IQ scores, and the (supposed) relationship between IQ and socioeconomic status (SES). In what follows, I will present several versions of the basic argument, and then attempt to show why not only are the arguments flawed as given, but also that no argument that uses the sorts of evidence these arguments use can possibly succeed in showing what they wish to show.

Briefly, the arguments start with a few pieces of empirical evidence that are then leveraged in an inappropriate way. The pieces of evidence are, roughly speaking, the following: (a) that there is a difference in SES between two groups; (b) that there is a difference in average IQ score between two groups; (c) that within each group, performance on IQ tests is a heritable trait; and (d) that within each group, IQ scores are correlated with SES. The latter two facts are then put to use in "explaining" the former facts, and it is here that conceptual errors and confusions come into play. The most basic problem, as we shall see, is that within-group heritability estimates cannot be used to explain differences observed *between* groups. After exploring this problem in some detail, two other major problems with the use of heritability in these cases will be briefly explored; namely, their failure to deal with the questions about the possibilities of changing environments, and their failure to deal with the possibilities of complex gene-environment interactions.

The Argument: From the Heritability of IQ to Race

Jensen, in his infamous 1969 article "How Much Can We Boost IQ and Scholastic Achievement?" managed to make just about every mistake possible in the use of human heritability estimates. The basic structure of Jensen's argument follows the argument structure alluded to above very closely. First, Jensen noted that there exist significant average differences in performance on IQ tests between different "races."[3] In this article, he was primarily concerned with those between black Americans and white (Caucasian) Americans. Next, Jensen noted that performance on IQ tests is largely heritable. From there, he observed that academic success tends to follow performance on IQ tests, and is associated with social success. The conclusion Jensen drew from this is that there are limits to the extent to which we can hope to alleviate differences in academic achievement, and therefore social success, between "racial" groups.

A quarter century later, Murray and Herrnstein, in their best-selling book *The Bell Curve* (1994), presented the following syllogism:

[1] If differences in mental ability are inherited, and [2] if success requires those abilities, and [3] if earnings and prestige depend on success, then [4] social standing (which reflects earnings and prestige) will be based to some extent on inherited differences among people. (Murray and Herrnstein 1994, 105)

They then attempt to defend this syllogism by trying to show that differences in mental ability are in fact "substantially heritable." The authors argue that IQ is a reasonable measure of mental ability; this argument is placed in the introduction and relies heavily on Jensen's *Bias in Mental Testing* (1980), a massive and misnamed tome in which he argues that there is no bias. Murray and Herrnstein then claim that current estimates of the heritability of IQ make the estimate they use, .6, likely to be on the low side, and that further, an estimate of .6 ± .2 will get them all they need and includes most recent estimates on the heritability of IQ (1994, 105–8). Most of part 2 of *The Bell Curve*, "Cognitive Classes and Social Behavior," is meant to demonstrate that earnings and prestige really do require those abilities revealed by high performance on IQ tests. The upshot is the claim that, indeed, social standing is based, to a rather large extent, on inherited differences among people (see for example chapter 21, "The Way We Are Headed"). At this point, all Murray and Herrnstein have claimed is that *within* a particular group, the high heritability of IQ, and the link between IQ and socioeconomic status means that SES will be based at least in part on something heritable. While even this result is deeply flawed (see "Forget about Race," below), had they left it at this, their book would likely have been far less controversial than it was—and it likely would have sold far fewer copies as well!

The more controversial aspect of the book lies in the two chapters that are devoted to showing that this result holds for the differences in economic success met with by different "racial populations" in the United States. Chapter 13, "Ethnic Differences in Cognitive Ability," is primarily about the differences in the mean IQ scores of black and white populations in the United States. The authors argue that the difference in mean black and white IQ scores cannot be accounted for by any of the following: by testing bias (1994, 285–86), by differing socioeconomic status (286–88), or by the historical legacy of slavery and continuing legacy of racism (I interpret the otherwise inexplicable discussion of the IQ scores of African blacks on 288–89 as their attempt to show this). There is a brief discussion of the past convergence of average IQ scores in black and white populations, which, they claim, has now stalled and may even be reversing itself (289–95). Murray and Herrnstein then conclude that while it is likely that there is an environmental component to the black/white average IQ differences in the United States, at least some of the difference must be genetic (288–89, 311).

The two arguments above, that given by Jensen and that given by Murray and Herrnstein, are clearly closely related. Indeed, in many ways, Murray and Herrnstein's argument is simply a longer version of Jensen's, one that attempts to deal with some of the flaws in, and objections raised to, that earlier piece. In what follows, I will argue that not only have Murray and Herrnstein not provided a particularly good defense of the thesis that genetic differences between "races" are responsible for the differences in average IQ scores in the current population of the United States, but that even framing the thesis in this way is deeply misleading. In short, the following will argue that whether or not current mean IQ score distributions are different between "races" in a way that is related to genetic differences is entirely irrelevant for explaining (in any important sense) those differences that exist or for thinking about what the future could hold.[4] The conceptual limitations of "heritability" make the sorts of predictions and explanations that surround the arguments based on IQ and "race" deeply flawed, perhaps to the extent of being entirely incoherent.

There are a number of other places where the arguments given by Jensen and those given by Murray and Herrnstein could be questioned. These include, but are by no means limited to: the problems with the evidence for the high heritability of performance on IQ tests, which include the problems involved with measuring heritability in natural populations more generally (see for example Bailey 1997); problems with the concept of IQ and its relationship to intelligence (see for example Lewontin et al. 1984); and problems with the concept of "race" as it is used in these arguments (see for example Bailey 1997; Cavalli-Sforza and Cavalli-Sforza 1995). For the most part, I am going to ignore these problems in what follows, and concentrate on the problems that are directly related to the relationship between the claimed findings in human genetics research and the claimed implications that these findings are supposed to have for predictions and explanations that matter to the sorts of social policies we adopt. I will start with the most basic of the problems faced by arguments of this sort; that is, the difficulty in moving from within-population data to between-population explanations. Next, I will move to progressively more complex difficulties, such as the inability of the data marshaled by these arguments to deal with changing environments, and the inability of the data to deal with the possibility of complex gene-environment interactions.

Within- and Between-Population Differences

A high heritability for some trait within a given population cannot be used to argue for a genetic etiology of differences for that trait *between* populations that experience different environmental distributions and/or that have different distributions of relevant genotypes. Indeed, the claim that because the heritability of trait is, say, .8, that .8 of the difference *between* the average phenotypes of two different populations can be accounted for by genetics is now a well-known fallacy. As Plomin et al. note, "[e]ven if heritability within each of two groups were 100 percent, the difference between the groups could be completely environmental in origin" (Plomin et al. 1990, 367). Consider, for example, height, which, in the samples from populations in the United States, has been estimated to have a heritability of about .9. While this does mean that differences in height are mostly genetic in the samples used to generate the estimate, it *cannot* be taken to mean that the differences in height *between* groups are mostly genetic. Note, for example, the relatively recent growth in average height of Japan's population—a spurt that, it is widely believed, is to be accounted for almost entirely by environmental reasons. Obviously, the claim that most of the differences in height between native Japanese and white citizens of the United States in, say, the early 1960s were genetic, because most of the differences in the samples from the United States could be accounted for genetically, would have been false.

A similar argument, by the way, holds true for molecular studies. Basically, it is easy to mistake mere statistical *associations* for a *causal* connection if one is not careful to properly partition one's samples. Hamer and Copeland develop an amusing example of some hypothetical, badly misguided researchers searching for the "successful use of selected hand instruments" (SUSHI) gene (hypothesized to be associated with chopstick usage) between residents in Tokyo and Indianapolis. Hamer and Copeland note that while you would be almost certain to find a gene "associated with chopstick usage" if you did this, the design of such a hypothetical study would be badly flawed. What would be likely to happen here is that a genetic marker associated with the heterogeneity of the group involved (Japanese versus Caucasians) would be found, and the heterogeneity of the group involved would independently account for the differences in the trait; in this case, there is a cultural tendency for more people who grow up in Japan than people who grow up in Indianapolis to learn how to use chopsticks. That is, growing up in Japan is the causally important factor in using chopsticks; having a certain genetic marker is only *associated* with chopstick use in a statistical way, and only because those people who grow up in Japan are *also* more likely to have the marker than those who grew up in Indianapolis. The genetic marker is in no way causally related to chopstick use! That the genetic marker ends up associated with chopstick use is therefore just an accident of the design (Hamer and Copeland 1998, 43; Bailey 1997 develops a similar example). For this reason, careful attempts to find genes associated with traits using current molecular genetics approaches should take care that the populations they study are as homogeneous as possible; this, it is thought, will tend to prevent spurious associations of the sort described above. Indeed, it is often argued that the best way to perform these studies is to do them within single families, where some of the sorts of genetic and cultural variables that might otherwise throw off the results will be minimized (see Hamer and Copeland 1998, 43; Hamer and Copeland 1994; and Hamer et al. 1993). While this makes the results the studies get less likely to be wholly spurious associations (as the SUSHI gene would be), it also makes them more limited with respect to the ability to be generalized to other contexts. That is, while using a narrowly selected homogeneous population is a good way to avoid spurious associations, any results that one gets are harder to generalize to, for example, populations, other genetic contexts, or other environments.

In any event, as was pointed out quite soon after the publication of Jensen's article, the experiences of black and white Americans in the United States are radically different, and there is no way to control for differences of environment between them. Jensen attempted to do so by controlling for income, but this is obviously inadequate. Below, I discuss the research done on the IQ scores of "caste-like" minorities. Briefly, though, even controlling for income, average IQs of the caste-like minority in countries where it is regarded badly are much lower than average; in populations that have emigrated to places where they are not recognized as a separate group, average IQs go up to the population average (see below on Ogbu's and de Vos's work on the Buraku in Japan). But more prosaically, the way in which income translates into economic and political power is at best mildly, or over the very long term. The relatively recent emergence of a black middle class in the United States cannot be taken to mean that blacks and whites with the same middle-class incomes have equal access to power resources, as, for example, at least many whites will have long-standing social ties that permit them access to far more or better information, favors, and privileges than at least many blacks at the same income level. I am thinking here of access to such things as medical care, real estate, and financial market information, where who you know is often thought to matter at least as much as how much you can pay.

But the basic point is that heritability estimates derived from one population, or even from each population individually, and used on differences in phenotypes between population groups in different environmental distributions are, technically, meaningless. Given that there are, at the heart of this issue, two very different populations whose members experience very different environments, it should be clear that heritability estimates are of no use whatsoever.

Murray and Herrnstein's attempts to deal with this problem are, as has been noted above, somewhat more sophisticated. They confront the issue directly when they note that the fact that "a trait is genetically transmitted in individuals does not mean that group differences in that trait are also genetic in origin" (298), and they even give an example about planting "two handfuls of genetically identical seed corn . . . one handful in Iowa, the other in the Mojave" (298), an example that Block traces back to Lewontin's 1970 response to Jensen 1969 (see Block 1995, 110). They even go on to note that the environment for black Americans has often been closer to the Mojave in their analogy, and that of white Americans closer to Iowa (298).

They then phrase the issue in the usual way. The claim is that either (1) all the differences in mean IQ scores between black Americans and white Americans are the result of there being an environment component favoring white Americans (genetic effects neutral), (2) there is both a genetic component favoring white Americans and an environmental component favoring white Americans, or (3) there is merely a genetic component favoring white Americans (environmental effects neutral). Block notes that a fourth possibility, all the environmental difference favoring whites but a genetic difference favoring blacks is generally excluded, as Murray and Herrnstein have done here (Block 1995, 101, 102). This is not, Block notes, merely a logical possibility, but one that serious attention should be paid to, if one is going to pay any attention to the debate at all. Indeed, the very few studies done on cross-racial adoptions have either pointed to no differences in IQ between "races" or, in some cases, a statistically insignificant advantage for blacks (see Lewontin et al. 1984, 127–28). As Block points out, average phenotypic differences between groups can be, and sometimes are, the opposite of what the average genetic differences would be in another range of environments.

Consider the case of skin color in, say, the nineteenth-century Spanish aristocracy and white, blue-eyed surfers in California in the 1970s, to pick a date before people started worrying quite so much about skin cancer! While the nineteenth-century Spanish aristocracy tanned well and easily, for social reasons they strove to keep out of the sun and remain as light-colored as possible. On the other hand, at least in the 1970s, surfers strove to keep their skins as dark as possible, despite tanning comparatively poorly. Given equal exposure to sun, it seems more than likely that the members of the nineteenth-century Spanish aristocracy would be rather darker than those surfers; however, it is at least very plausible that in fact many members of the nineteenth-century Spanish aristocracy were significantly lighter-skinned than many of the blue-eyed surfers in the 1970s. That is, the actual phenotypic difference could well have been in the opposite direction of that which "equal exposure to the sun" would generate. In any event, as will become clear, the issue is not so much which side of the debate is right, but whether the debate is a sensible way to deal with any of the issues it attempts to confront. In this sense, the limitation of possibilities is, as Block notes, worth noting more for its power to make the claim that all the difference is environmental seem like an "extremist hypothesis," than because that way of phrasing the question makes any sense within the context of arguments premised on broad-sense heritability (see Block 1995, 102).

Murray and Herrnstein admit that there is quite likely an environmental component to differences in mean IQ scores between black and white Americans. What they attempt to show, though, is that this component is unlikely to be able to account for the entirety of the difference that currently exists.

They initially put this difference at about 1.2 standard deviations, or something on the close order of 17 IQ points (Murray and Herrnstein 1994, 277–79), but later back off and go for a "low" estimate of 1 standard deviation, or some 15 IQ points. Given this, they argue that to explain a 1-standard-deviation difference in solely environmental terms, given a heritability of IQ of around .6, would mean assuming that the environmental mean of white Americans is better than the environmental mean of black Americans by some 1.58 standard deviations.[5] Assuming a normal (Gaussian) distribution, they argue that it is unlikely that the average environment of black Americans is really at the bottom 6th percentile of the distribution of environments of white Americans (299).[6]

There are a number of problems with this line of reasoning. Note for example that heritability estimates make no mention, and indeed *can* make no mention, of actual environmental conditions (see chapter 3). Hence, what it means for an environment to be, for example, "1.58 standard deviations" better or worse is, in this case, simply that it be that environment that makes that particular phenotypic variation disappear. From the standpoint of figuring out how different the environments would actually have to be in terms of actual environmental conditions to make the phenotypic variation in observed mean IQ scores disappear, knowing that it is "1.58 standard deviations" is quite useless. In other words, you need to answer the question of how "1.58 standard deviations" translates into actual environmental conditions, such as incomes of parents, number of books in the home, years of schooling of parents and children, degree and freedom of broad social acceptance, and so on, before you can make any sense of that number. In the phenomenon known as *canalization,* in certain environmental ranges, relatively large changes in actual environmental conditions lead to at most relatively small changes in resulting phenotypic values. It is in this range that the phenotype is said to be *canalized.* In other environmental ranges, outside the range of environments where the phenotype is canalized, relatively small changes in actual environmental conditions lead to relatively large changes in resulting phenotypic values (see figure 4.1). Knowing the broad-sense heritability of a trait

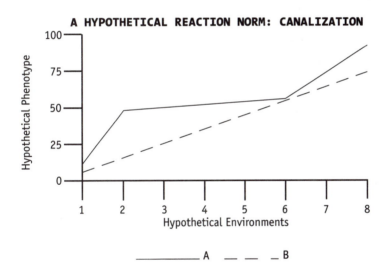

Data for Figure 4.1

Hypothetical phenotype scores for two hypothetical genotypes in eight hypothetical environments:

Environments/Genotype	1	2	3	4	5	6	7	8
A		10	48	50	52	54	56	75	90
B		5	15	25	35	45	55	65	75

Figure 4.1: A hypothetical reaction norm showing canalization. Notice that the trait corresponding to genotype A is highly canalized between environments 2–6, whereas genotype B shows no canalization.

within a population is useless if what one wants to know is how much one has to change an environmental variable to change a resulting phenotypic value. Given this, what it means for the environment of white Americans to be "1.58 standard deviations" better than that of black Americans is entirely opaque. In order to control for this, we would have to know rather more about how each of the various environmental differences affected the phenotypic differences in question for the various genotypes than we do in fact know, or have any way of finding out. We would need, in other words, to know the norms of reactions for various human geno-types in various complex social environments. Murray and Herrnstein, of course, ignore the issue entirely.

Perhaps even more significantly, it isn't at all clear why a normal (Gaussian) distribution should be assumed here. Indeed, it is far from obvious that any white Americans, even those in the bottom 6th per-centile of the environmental distribution of white Americans, experience an environment relevantly similar to that experienced by any black Americans. This is not to say that every black American's environment is worse than every white American's, just that they are not the same in many relevant ways. The environments of wealthy black Americans, for example, are undoubtedly markedly superior in many ways to those of very poor white Americans; however, even wealthy black Americans face an environment in which they are the target of racism (at least occasion-ally, often on an ongoing basis), in a way that poor white Americans sim-ply do not.[7] My argument here is that the environment faced by "Americans," then, cannot be well-ranked from "great" to "awful" in such a way that the different experiences of, for example, black and white Americans are amply accounted for. The effects of living as a member of an ill-thought of minority are such as to make the idea of a "normal" envi-ronmental distribution that could encompass both the experiences of black and white Americans in a sensible way seem hopeless.

Block, for example, notes that there is ample evidence that in at least some cases, the mere fact of being an oppressed minority affects such things as performance on IQ tests and resulting IQ scores in radical ways. He cites Ogbu's work on what happens when members of caste-like minorities emigrate to other societies. The Buraku, for example, an ill-thought-of group in Japan, have IQ scores 10–15 points lower than other Japanese, even controlling for socioeconomic status. Those differences in average IQ scores, however, vanish entirely in those Buraku who have emigrated to countries in which they are not recognized as a group dis-tinct and different from other Japanese (Block 1995, 113–44; see also de Vos 1992, 164–65). Given this observation, the United States's history as a racial state, and the continuing legacy of racism in the United States (see for example Omi and Winant 1994), it doesn't seem at all unreasonable to assume that environmental differences drive the entirety of the differences in average IQ scores. Indeed, Murray and Herrnstein note Ogbu's research and its implications, but then proceed to ignore it entirely in formulating their conclusions (1994, 307).[8]

Steele and Aronson's work on the interaction of stereotyping and testing should also be taken as a warning against interpreting the differences between "races" in mean performance on IQ tests as reflecting differences in "intelligence" per se. Steele and Aronson found that, for example, blacks who were told they were taking a diagnostic "intelligence" test significantly underperformed compared to blacks who were told it was not diagnostic of ability. Whites, on the other hand, performed equally well under both conditions. This obviously has serious implications for how the results of IQ tests are interpreted. Indeed, Steele and Aronson found that merely being asked to state one's race, irrespective of the description of the test, lowered the average scores of blacks, but not whites. Again, these results should inspire us to be extremely cautious in thinking about the way that different populations can respond differently to "the same" kinds of environments (Steele and Aronson 1995; see also Steele 1997, 1998).

Looking at the history of IQ scores in developed Western nations reveals that there is something deeply questionable about the line that Murray and Herrnstein take in *The Bell Curve*. There has been a gradual increase in the average IQ score in such nations, where it has been tracked at all (the so-called Flynn effect; see Block 1995, 124; Murray and Herrnstein 1994, 307–09). Block notes that the gap between the average IQ score in Holland in 1952 and 1982, a gap of some 21 points, must have been the result of environmental and not genetic changes in the Dutch. Any argument attempting to show that the genetic distribution of the Dutch changed radically between 1952 and 1982 would be implausible, to say the least. It seems, however, somewhat bizarre to claim that the average environment of the Dutch in 1992 was 2.21 standard deviations "better" than that in 1952—indeed, I think it is unclear what such a claim would even mean. Even worse, following Murray and Herrnstein's reasoning would lead us to conclude that the average Dutch environment of 1952 would be below the bottom 1.5 percent of the Dutch environmental distribution of 1982! However, I cannot see how to avoid being forced to draw absurd conclusions like these if we follow Murray and Herrnstein's reasoning about black and white environmental differences in America.[9]

Murray and Herrnstein, indeed, seem to realize that the Flynn effect makes something of a mess of their argument. Primarily, they take this effect as evidence that there "are things we do not yet understand about the relation between IQ and intelligence," things that "may be relevant for comparisons not just across times but also across cultures and races," and they also note that the Flynn effect should "caution against taking the current ethnic differences as etched in stone" (1994, 309). Again, though, after mentioning these problems they proceed to develop their own arguments as if these problems were not just solvable, which they provide no evidence for, but actually solved. In any event, given that we must be able to account for differences of at least 21 IQ points in wholly environmental terms, without having a clue what the environmental differences that drove the change actually were, it shouldn't strain our credulity at all to assume that the black/white difference in contemporary society is entirely environmental.

In saying, though, that the assumption that the differences are entirely environmental shouldn't strain our credulity, I certainly don't want to imply that we have any good evidence for such a claim either. We don't, in fact, even know enough about the way that genes interact with their contexts to produce complex human traits like intellectual ability to know if this is a sensible way to phrase the question. But we certainly have no evidence that the fact that the mean scores on IQ tests of black Americans are currently significantly lower than those of white Americans is in any way inevitable or immutable.

The Changing Environment and the Genetic

The argument against moving from within-population differences to explanations of between-population differences was explored in some detail above. I now wish to turn a slightly different point. As we saw in the last chapter and in the discussion of Cooper and Zubek's work on maze-running ability in rats (see above, and box 3.2 and figure 3.1), the high heritability of variation in a trait in one range of environments provides no evidence of its degree of heritability in different environmental ranges. Since the most natural way to attempt to modify an individual's academic achievement is through environmental interventions—interventions that will often result in the creation of new environmental conditions, a high heritability of performance on IQ tests, or academic achievement more generally in one environment—does not entail that, when attempts to modify the trait in question are carried out, there will remain a high heritability for the trait in question. Further, the high heritability of a trait, even within a range of environments, does not preclude the existence of large environmental effects as well. It was perhaps some combinations of these flaws in Jensen's reasoning that Lewontin was getting at when he noted that "the only way we could answer [the question posed in the title to Jensen's paper: 'How much can we boost I.Q. and academic achievement?'] would be to try to boost IQ and scholastic achievement . . . not . . . by asking . . . whether there is a genetic influence on IQ, because to be genetic is not to be unchangeable" (Lewontin 1993, 35). There are at least two senses of Lewontin's comments, both of which provide sharp critiques of Jensen's, as well as Murray and Herrnstein's, arguments. First, a weaker sense of this comment will be explored; that is, even assuming that the environment and the genes in question interact in an additive fashion, the argument doesn't hold. The stronger reading, which questions the additivity of the effects of the genetic and environmental influences, will then be laid out.

Koshland, in an editorial in *Science*, argued that recent findings involving the heritability of complex traits implied that "better schools, a better environment, better counseling and better rehabilitation will help some individuals but not all" (1987, 1445). By now, I hope it is obvious that by the very nature of the concept of heritability, no estimate for heritability *could* imply any such conclusion (no matter how impeccable the study or how high the estimated heritability turned out to be). The concept simply does not permit heritability estimates to be used in making judgments about what will happen in different environmental distributions. If anything counts as constituting a different environmental range, or a different distribution of the population within a range, I take it that "better schools, a better environment, better counseling and better rehabilitation" would be likely candidates.[10]

Jensen, however, had addressed this problem by assuming, in effect, that the effects of environment on IQ scores, across any relevant range of environments and genotypes, would be additive. Given this assumption, for any two genotypes, G1 and G2, if in any one given environment organisms of genotype G1 have a higher mean IQ score than organisms of genotype G2 by amount x, then within any other similar environments, organisms of genotype G1 will still have a higher mean IQ score than organisms of genotype G2, by the same amount x (see figure 4.2). So, while a better environment would help raise the scores achieved on IQ tests by people whose IQ scores were low, it would also help raise the scores achieved on IQ tests by people whose IQ scores were high. The *difference*, however, would remain, and according to Jensen, it is the difference that matters.

Jensen also argues briefly for a somewhat different conclusion—that intelligence cannot be very "plastic"—on both empirical and theoretical grounds (1982). Jensen claims that the low plasticity for intelligence

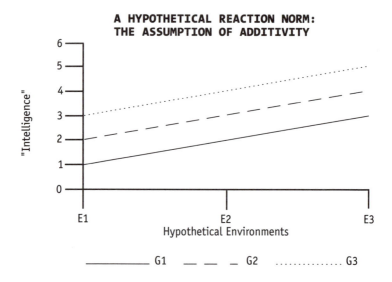

Data for Figure 4.2

Hypothetical phenotype scores for three hypothetical genotypes in three hypothetical environments:

Environment/Genotype	E1	E2	E3
G1	1	2	3
G2	2	3	4
G3	3	4	5

Figure 4.2: A hypothetical reaction norm displaying Jensen's assumption of additivity with respect to "intelligence" over various environments.

argues away from increased funding for education as a way of improving people, and toward "eugenic means" (1982, 1). Empirically, he takes as his main evidence the fact that programs to raise the performance of children on IQ tests have not met with much success.[11] But the conclusion he draws from this, that human intelligence isn't very plastic, is too strong. The proper conclusion to draw from the (claimed) failure of relatively short-term, more-or-less intensive academic programs to help children already identified as poor academic performers to perform much better on IQ and other evaluative tests is, I think, simply that such programs don't in fact help children already identified as poor performers perform much better. Whatever it is in the environment that is associated with variation on performance on IQ tests, *that* isn't it. Whether it is the sort of thing we can find and exploit, however, remains an open question—but, again, the only way of finding out is to keep trying, since no theoretical arguments either way will have much force, and the empirical evidence is spotty and mixed.

Indeed, there is good empirical evidence for some plasticity of performance on IQ tests. In the very adoption studies that Jensen, and Murray and Herrnstein, so love to cite as providing evidence for the high heritability of IQ, the performance on IQ tests of children adopted away from their biological parents was significantly greater than the performance on IQ tests of children who stayed with their biological parents (see Lewontin et al. 1984, 116ff, and Hamer and Copeland 1998, 219–23 for a summary of some of these results). Jensen's theoretical grounds for arguing against plasticity of intellectual ability are simply strange. Jensen claims that IQ measures something key to the survival of humans, and a "too-plastic malleability would give the organism little protection against the vagaries of its environment" (1982, 2). From the standpoint of the work done on the evolution of phenotypic plasticity and its relationship to fitness, however, this is a very odd claim to make indeed. Phenotypic plasticity is often what allows an organism to have a reasonably high fitness in various environments it may encounter, *not* something that generally prevents it from doing well (see Schlichting and Pigliucci 1998 and Pigliucci and Schlichting 1995). *If* performance on IQ tests proves to be a highly "plastic" trait, there would be no difficulty, in principle, of accounting for this. While we currently have little or no evidence one way or the other, nor any way of getting the evidence needed, stories that would relate the plasticity of performance on IQ tests to such phenomena as allometry or other constraints would be all too easy to tell (see chapter 3).

In any event, even granting the bold assumption of additivity, Koshland at least still got it wrong. The reason that Koshland's mistake is so serious in this context is that unlike Jensen, who despite his somewhat misleading title ("How Much Can We Boost IQ and Scholastic Achievement?") was really thinking about competitiveness, Koshland seems not to have been. No one believes that the trait in question, intellectual ability broadly construed, is *entirely* nonplastic. Given this, even if we assumed perfect additivity, which is an assumption we have no reason to make, changes in the environments *could* indeed help many people. Perhaps something like "competitiveness" *might* not be helped by the changes hinted at, but again, that's a different question. If "improved schools, environments, counseling and rehabilitation" succeeded in doing what they were supposed to, then even assuming that competitiveness remained unchanged, so many things would be helped that competitiveness would hardly seem to matter at all.

By this I mean that if, for example, the psychological torture associated with, say, mental illness is not entirely socially mediated, then, even if improving social systems such that everyone were a bit saner, and even saner by exactly the same amount wouldn't make anyone better off *comparatively*, it might still make a huge difference to the lives of those people at the bottom (more on this later).[12] Or again, even if Jensen's assumptions about the near-perfect additivity of performance on IQ tests were true, it might still be possible to boost "scholastic achievement" at least in some legitimate senses of the phrase, and perhaps even to boost it radically. If everyone's ability to do mathematical problems were boosted by the same amount, relative rankings as measured on open-ended math tests might well be unchanged, but, we can suppose, any number of people who couldn't balance their checkbooks before the boost would be able to do so after it. Some changes that don't change rankings don't matter; some do. There is often no obvious way to tell ahead of time what kind of change one is facing.

Again, though, Jensen, and certainly Murray and Herrnstein, are not concerned with abilities in general but with comparative advantages. Indeed, when discussing the Flynn effect Murray and Herrnstein note that while we might expect mean black American IQ scores to creep upwards with the Flynn effect, there is no reason to suppose that those of white Americans won't do so as well. "There seems" they note, no reason to suppose that the mean IQ scores of black Americans couldn't be raised 15 points or so through environmental changes but "also no reason to believe that white and Asian means can be made to stand still while the Flynn effect works its magic" (308).[13] The implication is that it is the gap that matters, and, given the implicit assumption of additivity, any changes that increase mean black American IQ scores will do the same for white American IQ scores. Thus the gap, and hence relative competitiveness, will remain unchanged. Murray and Herrnstein state that "at any point in time, it is one's position in the distribution [of IQ scores] that has the most significant implications for social and economic life as we know it" (309).

This claim should give raise to rather grave doubts; many people would read the statistics surrounding the current social inequalities as showing that, for example, the socioeconomic status (SES) of one's parents is a much more important predictor of one's eventual SES than one's performance on IQ tests (see Lewontin et al. 1984, 93–94). But that issue aside, even Murray and Herrnstein seem to have some doubts about the truth of these claims with respect to social standing in the United States as recently as the 1950s. They imply that at that time, "hard work" could make up for a general lack of raw intelligence and make one a useful, well-paid, and respected member of a community even if one wasn't particularly bright (see, for example, page 542, on "sweat equity" and getting ahead by hard work). Curiously, by 1997 Murray seems to have changed his mind about the very possibility or indeed wisdom of not particularly bright people being respected members of the community at all (see Murray 1997).

But competitiveness is a rather tricky concept more generally. Radically boosting everyone's "scholastic achievement" an equal amount might or might not improve the competitiveness of the disadvantaged groups. For some tasks, it seems clear, once a certain ability level has been reached, further "achievements" are simply irrelevant. For tasks like these, a large increase in everyone's ability could well result in everyone, or far more people anyway, being equally qualified, despite the fact that there were still in some sense absolute differences in abilities between them. For other tasks, of course, it might well be the case that more is always better, as far as abilities are concerned. But until we know rather more about the tasks at hand, and what it means for "scholastic achievement" to be boosted or abilities gained, it is hard to know what to make of this argument. The argument seems, indeed, to have been kept at too abstract a level for it to achieve its ends. Even assuming additivity, then, the argument is deeply problematic.

The above discussion was premised on the assumption of additivity—an assumption that there was little reason to have any faith in. Indeed, as was stressed in chapter 3, contemporary research into the plasticity of various traits has tended to point away from linearity and toward more complex interactions between genes and their contexts; it seems that the "topologies" of norms of reaction can be expected to be quite complex (see for example figures 3.5–3.7). However, once the assumption that average IQ scores will respond to environmental changes in a straightforwardly linear way is abandoned, it becomes impossible to make *any* meaningful claims about the relationship between a high broad-sense heritability of the trait and the likely effects of environmental intervention.

If additivity fails to hold in some ranges of possible environments, predicting what will happen in a new environment to a trait like performance on IQ tests, based on broad-sense heritability in some environment, is, again, obviously impossible. It might be thought that merely shifting the distribution of environments within the current set of existent environments would get around some of these problems, and that the sorts of changes alluded to by, for example, Koshland—better schools, a better environment, and the like—are really of this sort. But again, without any additional information on what environmental variables affect IQ scores and how, a high heritability in one environmental distribution does not point toward much of anything regarding the likely effects of environmental distributions that are subsets of the previous environmental distribution.

Consider again the example of Cooper and Zubek's work on maze-running ability in rats (see above and previous chapter). In an environmental distribution such that both strains of rats, "maze-bright" and "maze-dull," were distributed across all three types of environments, "impoverished," "ordinary," and "enriched," at equal frequencies, both heritability and environmentality would emerge as sizable components of an analysis of variance. This, again, is because there is a tendency for maze-bright rats to be, on average, better maze-runners, and a tendency for maze-running ability to increase as available environmental stimulation increases. If the only information available was the broad-sense heritability of maze-running ability, it would remain unclear what effects various environmental changes would have. This would include changes that didn't create new environmental ranges but merely shifted environmental distributions; that is, that put more of the rats of each type in, say, the enriched environment and fewer rats of each type in, the impoverished environment. Without information about the way the different strains of rats respond to various different environments—without, that is, the norms of reaction—it would be impossible to predict what even changes of that sort would result in. Knowing the norms of reaction, of course, we can predict that radical shifting of the environmental distributions toward the ordinary environment would tend to increase heritability, decrease environmentality, and generally increase the variance in the trait in question. This is because we know that it is only in the ordinary environment that the two strains of rats show a clear difference in maze-running ability. And, as we saw above, radically shifting the distribution away from the ordinary environments and toward the impoverished and enriched environments would tend to increase environmentality and decrease heritability. Obviously, these results are not predictable from the broad-sense heritability of the trait in the initial distribution.

As there is, at this time, no reason to suspect that whatever environmental and genotypic differences affect differences in performance on IQ tests do so in an additive way, it seems reasonable to treat the assumption of additivity with some skepticism. Given this, all attempts at predicting what effects changing various social or political policies would have on the distribution of IQ scores in various populations should be treated with at least an equal degree of skepticism. We just don't know how to move from the current data to predictions about the effects of possible educational policies or shifts in resources.

Gene-Environment Interactions: Genetic Differences and Differing Responses to the Environment
Both Jensen's and Murray and Herrnstein's arguments rely on there being a statistically significant difference between the genotypic distributions of black Americans and white Americans with respect to those genes that are related to performance on IQ tests. However, *if* there is a genetic difference between various "races" that affects performance on IQ tests,[14] then which conditions are best for developing those abilities that lead to high performance on IQ tests may vary as well. The best conditions for developing a trait like high performance on IQ tests in a population with one genetic distribution may be very different from those with another. Recall that, for example, different commercial strains of laboratory rats responded differently to different learning regimes, such as massed versus spread-out trial speed, with some learning faster under one sort of regime and others learning faster in other regimes.[15]

In general, one might think that arguments about genetic differences influencing performance on things like IQ tests would be faced with serious problems of this sort. If they assume a large average genetic difference to account for some phenotypic difference, they are faced with the problem that different genotypes do not in general respond to different environments in the same way. Recall Dobzhansky and Spassky's work on the viability of larval *Drosophila* (fruit flies) in different temperatures discussed in the last chapter (see figures 3.5–3.7). There we saw that there is no best temperature for every genotype: some respond well to relatively high temperatures, some to relatively low temperatures, some to middle temperatures, and some even had multiple peaks; that is, there was a "local minimum" at the middle temperature tested. Given this, the claim that there is going to be some one type of environment that will maximize the phenotypic score of organisms of *any* given genotype looks very hard to support. It may be in principle possible to get around this difficulty; however, it must at least be dealt with, something Murray and Herrnstein, for example, utterly fail to do or even attempt. Again, the claim that there must be some uniformly best environment for all genotypes—that is, some environment that will maximize the phenotypic result of any given genotype—is just plain false. If there is a statistically significant difference in genotypic distributions relevant to performance on IQ tests between black and white Americans, this problem alone would undermine any arguments to the fixed nature of current rankings.

"Forget about Race": SES, IQ, and Molecular Studies

Turning our attention away from the very controversial work done on the relationships among genetics, race, intelligence, and socioeconomic status, (SES), we can ask what people who have steered clear of the specific problems associated with arguments about "race" have argued for, and what the research they cite might actually support. In some cases, the arguments are very similar, both in style and conclusion, to those discussed above with respect to differences supposedly associated with "race." The authors in these cases claim that since it is known that "intelligence" is basically genetic, there isn't a whole lot that can be done about inequalities in society, and schools should stop trying to help the not-very-bright students who aren't going to get much better anyway. These arguments will be dealt with first; if the above arguments on the inability of heritability estimates to help us understand differences in the average SES of various "races" were convincing, disposing of these arguments will prove relatively quick. I will then turn toward contemporary molecular studies. In at least some of these cases, the claims for what has been found are far more cautious, and the policy implications (indeed, even the implications for further research) much vaguer. Again, the criticisms will follow much of the work laid out in chapter 3, applying the theoretical arguments developed there about molecular findings in the human case to this specific instance.

Socioeconomic Status, Intelligence, and Heritability (Again)
To approach the arguments about the relationship between the "naturalness" or inevitability of socioeconomic status and the heritability of IQ, *The Bell Curve* is once again as good a place to start as any. While the above section concentrated on claims in the book that regarded "race" (as did most of the media attention and reviews), most of the book isn't about "race" at all. The syllogism given above was *mainly* about differences in society generally, not between "ethnic" groups. Murray makes the point even more plainly in his "IQ Will Put You in Your Place" (1997), where he writes that if we had several hundred nearly ideal families and raised a bunch of children in them, rather than most of them doing well as we might expect,

> the bright children from such families will do well in life—and the dull
> children will do poorly. Unemployment, poverty, and illegitimacy will

be almost as great among children from even these fortunate families as they are in the society at large—not quite as great, because a positive family background does have some good effect, but almost, because IQ is such an important factor. (1997, 1)

What conclusion does Murray think should be drawn from this? He writes:

Inequality is too often seen as something that results from defects in society that can be fixed by . . . more active social programs, or better schools. It is just not so. (3)

Given their contention that IQ is largely genetic, Murray and Herrnstein (1994) argued that the direct link between IQ and SES meant that there wasn't a whole lot of room for "improving" the SES of those less well-off through education (chapter 17). While they note that "moving a child from an environment that is the very worst to the very best" may make a difference that is "considerable" even given "a heritability of .6," they argue that most changes won't be that radical, and in any event "such changes are limited in their potential consequences when heritability so constrains the limits of environmental effects" (109).

In a similar vein, Goodhart argues from the high heritability of IQ to the conclusion that since "differences really are inborn, there is no use forcing children beyond their natural capacities" (1994, 50). He implies that the claim that "extra resources should be devoted to children with these "special needs," rather than being used to enable those who are already doing well to do even better" is badly misguided, and that "a selective system . . . picking out those who will benefit from being fully stretched, with the rest going to schools to make the best of the abilities they do possess" would give "the best results" (50). In an interview with Seligman in the *National Review*, Murray stated that based on what was known about IQ, "most people are not smart enough to profit from an authentic college education," so policies to permit "universal college education" "wouldn't be" a "good policy idea" (Murray and Seligman 1997).

The conclusions these authors reach are misguided for very much the same reasons that the above arguments (focused though they were on "race') were misguided. Knowing the heritability of performance on IQ tests (or any other trait, for that matter) without knowing the reaction norms for the trait given the genes and environments associated with it simply does not permit one to make any judgments about how different environments would influence the performance on IQ tests of given individuals. Do the oft-cited "failures" of programs like Head Start to make massive and long-lasting improvements in performance on IQ tests (see

Murray and Herrnstein 1994, chapter 17; Jensen 1982) imply anything about the "plasticity" of intelligence? Not really—to find about the reaction norms we would have to know far more about the genotypic makeup of the populations involved. Would "failures" of the sort cited have anything to say about the modifiability of performance on IQ tests more generally? If they do, it is only that in the populations studied, you can't make a huge difference with a program that lasts for a couple hours a day, runs for a year or so, and starts relatively late in life. This may be an interesting result, but it obviously has very little to do with genetic explanations for variations in human intelligence.

The Cautions of the Molecule
There are many questions that could be considered when thinking about recent and projected work in finding genes "associated" with intellectual ability. Some of these are: (a) Can it be done *in principle*? (b) Is it being done well now? (c) If successful, what would it show (immediately) about the relationship between genetics and intellectual functioning in humans? (d) What implications would this have for thinking through issues surrounding the relationship of intelligence to social policy? (e) What directions for future research would it point toward? and (f) What implications might the finding of *that* future research have for thinking through social policy issues?

There have been two sorts of associations found between forms of genes and "intelligence," or tests purported to measure intelligence. An example of one form has already been discussed at some length in chapter 2: genes associated with severe mental disabilities. As we saw with PKU, genetic errors associated with metabolic disturbances, for example, can have profound effects on intellectual functioning. These cases are uncontroversial and also unhelpful from a policy standpoint. The best one can say is that more work is necessary, at the biochemical and medical end of things as well as at the political and social levels, to try to alleviate the human suffering that such diseases cause. I think that this is quite uncontroversial. It is certainly possible to argue about methodological questions, such as whether one should concentrate on the gene end of things or the phenotypic end of things, but these are not so much arguments about what is in principle possible as arguments about the best places to put scarce research dollars. But these cases obviously have few implications for intellectual functioning in the "normal" range. Hamer and Copeland draw one implication from the huge numbers of genes that, when they go wrong, interfere with the development of normal intelligence; namely, that the large number of genetic diseases associated with intellectual problems "offer a glimpse into how complicated the search" for genes associated with normal intellectual functioning will be, and for that matter how complicated a thing normal intellectual functioning *is* (1998, 223–31, 234–35).

The other sort of association searched for is that between high performance on tests meant to measure intelligence and particular forms of genes. At this time, the only association that has not been retracted yet was found by Plomin's team (see Chorney et al. 1998). They claim to have found a gene that accounts for some 2 percent of the variance in "g" (so-called general intellectual ability) of their test subjects (Chorney et al. 1998, 159). As was noted in the last chapter, molecular genetics studies that do little or nothing to elucidate the biochemical pathways that the gene is involved in can, and often do, show associations between forms of genes and complex traits. What they can't do is say much about the relationship these have to each other. Finding an association is not the same as finding a causal relationship, nor even an association which will hold in other contexts; we noted in the last chapter that a gene that is said to account for "about 10 percent" of the variation in novelty seeking (as Hamer and Copeland would have it; see 1998, 46) may do so only in some contexts; in different environments or in other genetic contexts, such a genetic variation may cease to be associated with any variations in novelty-seeking behaviors at all. The same is obviously true of alleles of genes associated with high intelligence. In other contexts, the same allele of the gene could have no effect, or the opposite one, on the trait in question. When Chorney et al. argue that "if the QTL [quantitative trait loci] . . . operates continuously throughout the distribution, the average effect of the allele would be an increase of about 4 IQ points" (1998, 164), the "if" should be taken very seriously indeed. We have no idea if the "quantitative trait locus" model is a good one for complex human traits (for a discussion of how very different mechanistic arrangements can yield the same sorts of quantitative data, see Pigliucci and Schlichting 1997, Schlichting and Pigliucci 1995). We have no idea if the allele associated with the discovery "operates continuously" throughout the contemporary distribution of genetic contexts. We also have no good way of finding out. Recall again that even in cases where the trait is not under "direct" genetic control, it will be possible to find associations of this sort if one looks for them. What to make of those associations is the real question, and it remains an open one.

However, we might ask if these (purported) discoveries point in interesting directions for future research. That is, perhaps finding the gene itself is of little interest, but it might *lead* to research programs that would yield interesting results. Perhaps they might, but some glimpse at how difficult such programs might be in humans can be seen, again, by looking at the literature attempting to make sense of the molecular genetics findings regarding relatively simple plants and relatively simple traits. (For one interesting attempt to unravel some of the significance of molecular genetics finding in a broader context, see Pigliucci and Schmitt, 1999; Pigliucci, et al. 1999a; Pigliucci et al. 1999b; Schmitt et al. 1999, and citations therein.) Even where one has full control of one's experimental subjects, and can perform, for example, gene knockout experiments at will, figuring out how particular genes are causally related to particular traits turns out to be far from trivial (see also Schlichting and Pigliucci 1998 for a general discussion of the problems involved in successfully integrating and understanding the relationships between developmental and evolutionary biology).

It should be obvious by now that what we *really* want to know in order to make policy decisions about spending education dollars and attempting to modify people's environments are the reaction norms for the genes and suites of genes, if such there be, involved with those aspects of human intellectual functioning that we care about, in those environments that we can recognize and modify.[16] Only these would permit us to make sensible policy decisions based on biological data. But again, without access to experimental subjects where the genotypes and environments can be simultaneously controlled, it is hard to see how such reaction norms could, even in principle, be generated. Without them, we must look elsewhere for guidance in formulating policy decisions.

Conclusion: Policy, Race and IQ, Genes, and Heritability

Given all the problems noted above, it should be clear that any attempt to argue from the high heritability of a trait like performance on IQ tests to suggestions that certain classes of policy changes would be ineffectual requires, at the very least, a large number of (rather bold) auxiliary assumptions. In particular, arguments in the style of Jensen's and Murray and Herrnstein's, which purport to show that the high heritability of IQ has some link to the current social and economic inequalities faced by different "races" in contemporary society, require a number of assumptions that are rarely mentioned and never appropriately defended.

What are these assumptions? As we have seen, it would need to be clear that performance on IQ tests was more than trivially heritable in some large range of contemporary environments and populations. Further, it would need to be shown that there was a statistically significant difference between various so-called races in the distribution of those genes that influence performance on IQ tests, and that these genes had effects that were predictable and generally additive. That is, the genes would have to interact with their contexts in a predictable and additive way, both in terms of their response to environmental changes and epistatic (gene-gene) effects, including the problems involved in the possibility that part of what is going on is a kind of nondirect coding for emergent properties. It would be necessary to show that all the different possible, or at least actually available, genotypes responded to environmental changes in much the same way, or that for some reason or another environmental changes were impossible (for more on this topic, see chapter 10). It would be necessary to show that socioeconomic status really did depend on these traits and on the relative ranking of them. If it were clear that all these assumptions were true, the argument would at least be able to get off the ground, though it would still be problematic. Far from it being the case that these assumptions are clearly true, many of them are highly questionable, and for some of them, especially those involving the relationships between the environments, the genes, and the traits in question, there is absolutely no evidence for them nor any way of gathering evidence for them. As it stands, then, the entirety of the arguments toward purported links between the high heritability of performance on IQ tests, differences in mean IQ scores between various "races," and differences in mean SES, should be discounted in their entirety.

The somewhat less-publicized claims about the relationship between high heritability and social policies *within* populations should also be discounted, for much the same reasons. Despite the claims of a few proponents, we have no good reason to believe that human intelligence isn't at least rather "plastic," and some reasons to think it might be. We have no good reason to think that the genes and environments involved all work in an additive fashion. And finally, we have no good reason to think that education policy should depend on which side of this empirical debate about the plasticity of intelligence, or the additive nature of the genes involved, is right.

Studies that purport to find genes associated with intelligence cannot be taken to support the assumptions made by those who link the high heritability of performance on IQ tests to particular social policies. Without knowing more about the reaction norms and other context-dependent behaviors of the genes, such assumptions as additivity and low plasticity remain entirely unwarranted. Nor is finding a form of a gene associated with some particular form of a trait in some population at some time the same as understanding the causal pathways between the genetics and the phenotypes in question. Such studies *may* provide the beginnings of a start into understanding, for example, the development of intellectual abilities in humans. However, fulfilling such promises will probably prove to be harder than most of the publicity around such findings might imply.

Where we lack biological data that is relevant to policy decisions about, for example, education, we must look to other sources for inspiration and to other kinds of evidence. Making use of bad, misleading, and/or irrelevant data in formulating our policy decisions is likely worse than having none at all. But in fact, we do have some relevant data. Research into effects of various kinds of educational policies is more than possible—it's being done, and far more could be done. Such studies would be a far better place to look to for information about the effects of possible educational policies than is contemporary human genetic research.

CHAPTER 5
CRIMINALITY AND VIOLENCE: THE BRAIN AND THE GENE

Crimes and Individuals

I f a small number of individuals are responsible for a large percentage of the violence and criminal behavior in a society, then preventing the crimes caused by most of these individuals would have a large impact on the rates of violence and crime in that society. If these individuals could be picked out, preferably early in their criminal careers, or, better yet, before their criminal careers had started, and could be prevented from committing (more) crimes, the rates of violence and crimes more generally could be quite efficiently reduced. And if violence and criminality are the result of genetic, and more generally biological, predispositions, then, the argument goes, it should be possible to do so.

This, in a nutshell, is the argument that lies behind much research into the genetic and biological bases for violent and criminal behavior. In his brief survey of the state of the current research into the biological bases of criminal behavior, Gibbs notes that one of the most consistent finding of social scientists interested in crime and violence is that "a very small number of criminals are responsible for most of the violence" and crimes (Gibbs 1995, 102). That in one study, for example, some 6 percent of the males studied committed roughly 70 percent of the violent crimes, is taken, Gibbs notes, as evidence that "[p]reventing just a small fraction of adolescent males from degenerating into chronic violent criminals could thus make a sizable impact on the violent crime rate" (1995, 102). Given current research into the brain chemistry, genetics, and biological markers of criminality, combined with current thinking in sociology, Gibbs notes that the notion that one "might be able to assemble a complicated model that can scientifically pick out those who pose the greatest threat of vicious attack seems to be gaining currency" (1995, 107). Indeed, some researchers are already suggesting that society "must identify high-risk persons at an early age and place them in treatment programs *before* they have committed" any crimes (Jeffery, quoted in Gibbs 1995, 107). Once research has shown that a person is, for biological reasons, likely to commit crimes and hence medically ill, another researcher suggests, they should be treated as medically ill, and treatment, if available, "should be mandatory" (Fishbein, quoted in Gibbs 1995, 107). If no treatment is available, then the potential recidivist criminal "should be held indefinitely" (Fishbein, quoted in Gibbs 1995, 107). Of course, currently even the best biological markers of criminality have very high "false positive" rates—that is, most people with the markers associated with criminality will never commit a serious crime (see Gibbs 1995, 102). The hope that future research will result in more reliable markers of criminality being found, however, seems unrelated to the enthusiasm researchers have for using the their current list of markers in a bid for the prediction and control of violent and criminal behavior (see Gibbs 1995, 107).

This story characterizes both the threat and the promise of research into the genetic and biological bases of violent and criminal behavior. The promise is that the small number of men who will commit the vast majority of crimes will be easily identified early in their criminal careers, if not before the start of them, and will be treated or at least removed from society. The most obvious threat is that biological markers for criminality, with their very high false positive rates, will be used to identify "potential" criminals for mandatory medical intervention. A more subtle threat is brought out by what the story *doesn't* talk about, such as the radically different rates of violent crime cross-culturally. Violence and criminality is taken to be an individual problem, and the solution to high rates of crime and violence in a society is taken to lie in modifying individuals, medically or otherwise, in a way internal to the individuals in question. This sort of analysis is very popular; Wilson and Herrnstein (1985), for example, give a radically individualistic analysis of the causes of crime, both in their rational choice theory of crime (see chapter 2, "A Theory of Criminal Behavior") and in their biological correlates analysis (see chapter 3, "Constitutional Factors in Criminal Behavior"). However, this sort of individualistic account ignores the way individuals are shaped by the society they live in, and it fails to deal with what must be at least most of the cause of the differing crime rates between, for example, major cities in

Western Europe and major cities in America. In what follows, the major research strategies that attempt to discover biological, and especially genetic, bases of criminal behavior will be explored with an eye toward these sorts of threats and promises.

Genes and Violence: Heritability and Evolutionary Stories

Studies into the genetic basis of criminal and violent behaviors follow several basic trends. The broad-sense heritability of criminal behavior has been estimated by adoption and twin studies. These studies look for correlations between parents and siblings with respect to criminal behavior, sometimes keeping the criminally violent and crimes of property separate, but often not. Other approaches to studying the genetic bases of criminal behavior include a sort of sociobiological storytelling, where what is to be explained is the existence of genes for what we now consider criminal behavior. Lastly, occasionally a very specific biological problem will be suspected of being correlated with criminal behavior, and standard methods of linkage analysis and direct sequencing will be used to find the genetic cause of the disorder. Sometimes, aspects of the specific biochemical pathway from the gene(s) involved to the disorder can even be elucidated. In any event, in this way the gene(s) involved can be shown to be associated with the criminal behavior insofar as the original biological problem was so associated.

In the next two sections the basic methods, and some of the results of the first two of these techniques will be explored; that is, sociobiological storytelling about criminality and violence as well as the traditional ways of estimating broad-sense heritability as applied to criminality and violence. Also, I will at least hint at some of the links among these methods. These sorts of studies are, in effect, studies of people who can be thought of as within the ordinary range of criminality and violence. Those studies that concentrate on specific genetic "errors" and linkage analysis will be covered in the next section, as it is often thought that it is these individuals who represent those criminals with the highest rescidivism rates.

A Framework: Heritability and Sociobiology
Studies of the heritability of criminality and violent behavior have been conducted since at least the turn of the century. Charles Davenport (1866–1944) firmly believed both criminality and violence to be heritable (although with many modern researchers, he apparently believed them separate traits; see Kevles 1985, 46–47, 62). Indeed, the influence of Davenport's eugenic theories was great enough, and his arguments

for the heritability of criminality apparently convincing enough, that in the first decades of the twentieth century fifteen or so states enacted laws that made criminals subject to involuntary sterilization (Kevles 1985, 100ff.).

In the hereditarian atmosphere of those times, Davenport and his ilk needed little other than a theoretical framework that *permitted* the inheritance of traits like criminality and violence and the observation that criminality often ran in families for their claims to look powerful. While Lombroso's theory of atavism as the key to criminality (see below) sits poorly with Davenport's separation of thievery and violence as separate *types* of activity (see Kevles 1985, 46), both provided a theoretical background, generally involving "primitiveness," that explained why there should be violence and criminality at all (see Gould 1981, 122ff., and below). The theories could also account for how such "primitive" and "atavistic" traits could get to the modern world unchanged. Davenport, for example, was a radical Mendelian, and claimed Mendelian inheritance for nearly every trait he studied (see Kevles 1985, 48ff.). What mattered to the studies of the heritability of criminality was that there were explanations for both why such traits would exist at all and for mechanisms for those traits being passed from generation to generation.

In a similar way, Harpending and Draper's rather boldly speculative exploration of the sociobiological roots of both violent and nonviolent behavior speaks of two broad "reproductive strategies" humans could pursue, and which, they claim, different populations of humans actually do pursue or did pursue during the relevant bits of evolutionary history (Harpending and Draper, in Moffitt and Mednick 1988). One of the strategies, they claim, leads to more broadly antisocial behavior such as rape, child abandonment, dishonesty, and violence. The other broad strategy, they claim, leads to lives built around a sort of happy domesticity, including long-term monogamous pairing, shared parental child-rearing, openness and honesty, and an aversion to violence. Their basic claim is that in some social settings, such as traditional hunter-gatherer societies, being a good provider and able to guilelessly take part in social activities is evolutionary selected for, and being antisocial actively selected against (see 296–97); in other social settings, such as early gardening communities, being antisocial is selected for, as successful violent competition and lying result in the most successful reproductive strategies (see 298–301). The split, they claim, follows the split between "father-absent" and "father-present" societies—or more broadly, between those societies where males compete with each other for access to women and those in which males spend their time provisioning for their own offspring (294,

301). The payoff to this piece of evolutionary storytelling is that genes for both antisocial and social types may well abound, and individual differences would depend on from which of these broad types most of one's genes for those social/antisocial traits emerged (305). Once again, there is a background story for why traits we in the civilized Western world disapprove of exist at all, and the traditional mechanisms for getting those traits to us.

Heritability Studies: Criminality and/or Violence
Early theories of the genetic basis of criminality and violence tended to conflate the two. Lombroso's atavistic throwbacks were supposed to be both criminal and violent by nature (see Wilson and Herrnstein 1985, 72ff.). Recent studies, though, have tended to separate crimes of violence from crimes of property, as well as habitual offenders from occasional criminals. In brief, several twin and adoption studies have pointed toward violent behavior and crimes of property not being, in general, related, and have pointed toward crimes of property as having a much clearer genetic component. Also, several studies seem to hint that insofar as there is a genetic component to the criminality of habitual offenders, it has a different etiology from those on the more "ordinary" part of the spectrum.

In the case of all criminal behavior, twin studies are thought to point toward a high degree of heritability, with an estimate of heritability around .5 as the average, but with some studies getting numbers as high as .6–.8. Adoption studies, though, have tended to point toward rather lower numbers, usually generating heritability estimates of somewhat under .4 (DiLalla and Gottesman 1991, 125–26; Plomin et al. 1990, 380–81, and 394–95; Mednick and Kandel, in Moffitt and Mednick 1988, 122). It is also the adoption studies that are said to point most obviously toward a different etiology for violent crimes and property crimes. Indeed, several adoption studies are seen as pointing toward there being a genetic component to property but not to violent crimes (see DiLalla and Gottesman 1991). The lack of a genetic basis for variation in violent or aggressive behavior, at least in the normal range of behaviors, is supported by what little observational data exists on violent behavior in twins, which, it is claimed, also show no genetic influence on ordinarily aggressive behavior (see Plomin et al. 1990, 387). On the other hand, several researchers have claimed that forms of abnormally aggressive behavior do seem to have a genetic component. Several studies, it is claimed, point toward something called "aggressive conduct disorder" in juvenile delinquents having a genetic component, as well as perhaps being related to antisocial tendencies in adults (see DiLalla and Gottesman 1991; Plomin et al. 1990, 381;

Plomin et al. 1997, 210–15). As always, it is important to keep in mind both the technical limitations of heritability estimates and the problems with generating accurate estimates in human populations (see chapter 3).

Finding Causes: The Dream of Prevention through Recognition

Much of the hope surrounding the study of the biological and genetic bases of criminal behavior and violence has been in the promise of prediction and control of criminal and violent behavior. The hope is that some set of techniques will allow the discovery of individuals who are likely or predisposed to commit crimes or to be violent before they actually do so. At least, the hope is that some set of techniques will permit one to predict which criminals are likely to go on to commit more crimes. In Lombroso's theory of criminality, which was popular through the turn of the century, criminal types displayed their criminality through biological markers, as well as self-imposed stigmata such as tattoos. Recent work in tracking down the genetic markers for MAOA deficiency can be viewed as a similar search for markers.[1] But whether past or present, the central aspect of these claims is that there are violent or criminal types and that these violent or criminal types of people are "marked" in a way that permits them to be identified irrespective of their actions in the world.

Lombroso's influential theory of the biological basis of criminality was based on the idea that criminals were "atavisms," throwbacks to an earlier, less "civilized" sort of person (see Gould 1981, 122ff., and Lewontin et al. 1984, 53–54). Lombroso wrote of such people that "we may think that he was born a criminal because he was born a savage" (Lombroso, quoted in Gould 1981, 125). As throwbacks to earlier types, they could be readily identified by certain physical traits, such as "a heavy and developed jaw, projecting [eye] ridges, an abnormal and asymmetrical cranium . . . projecting ears . . . a crooked or flat nose" (Lombroso, quoted in Lewontin et al. 1984, 53). Further, Lombroso noted such features as "relatively long arms . . . low and narrow forehead . . . diminished sensitivity to pain" and the "inability to blush" (Gould 1981, 125, 129–30). Atavistic criminal types also displayed their nature through tattooing, which reflected both their "insensitivity to pain" and their "atavistic love of adornment" (Gould 1981, 132).

With these biological markers in hand, Lombroso and his followers felt fit to make judgments about the likelihood that an individual was a criminal. Gould cites various court cases in which Lombroso and his colleagues, acting as expert witnesses in trials, provided evidence that the accused was of a "criminal type," and hence, we are to suppose, more likely to have committed the crime than would otherwise have been the case (see Gould 1981, 137–39). The Italian army apparently took Lombroso's recommendations seriously enough to screen its recruits for the criminal types most likely to kill their commanding officers, rejecting those with the physiological traits supposedly associated with this practice (Gould 1981, 136). While neither Lombroso nor his supporters argued explicitly for the arrest, jailing, or isolation of these criminal types before they'd committed an offense, they did argue for the "pre-screening of children so that teachers might prepare themselves and know what to expect from" such children (Gould 1981, 136). In Lombroso's words, teachers ought to expect "scholastic and disciplinary shortcomings" from such children and channel them into "careers more suited to their temperament" (Lombroso, quoted in Gould 1981, 136–38).

These biological types were, if not actually destined to commit crimes, then at least quite likely to, given anything like the right circumstances. Criminal types were "born to evil" and all social responses to crime "break as against a rock" when faced with these atavistic types (Lombroso, quoted by Gould 1981, 139). There followed from this a theory of criminal justice, namely that the punishment meted out for a crime should be tailored not to the nature of the crime but to the nature of the criminal. Ferri, a student of Lombroso's, wrote that "[p]enal sanctions must be adapted . . . to the personality of the criminal" rather than to "the objective gravity of the crime" (Ferri 1911, quoted in Gould 1981, 141). Some noncriminal people committed violent or criminal acts for understandable reasons, and shouldn't be punished too harshly, even for quite serious offenses; others were born criminals and should be put away for a very long time, or even forever, for even quite trivial offenses (Gould 1981, 141). Born criminal types were, by their very nature, dangerous and incapable of learning, and hence should be locked away from civilized society at the slightest excuse.

The argument here—that it is the nature of the criminal that is the issue, and hence that by divining criminal nature one can control crime[2]—continues to exercise a firm hold on the imagination of at least some researchers and policy makers today. Moffitt and Mednick claim, in the preface to a collection of essays sponsored by NATO, that "social and environmental variables cannot explain" those whose "criminal careers" start early and continue throughout life (Moffitt and Mednick 1988, preface, xiii). Being able to recognize those "5% of males [who] commit over 50% of criminal offenses" would allow one, they claim, to "dramatically reduce our growing crime rate" by "intervention directed at these relatively few individuals" (Moffitt and Mednick 1988, preface, xiii; see also Gibbs 1995, esp. 102, 107).

Research into the link between violence and MAOA deficiency in humans is said by at least one researcher involved to have somewhat similar consequences. Breakefield is quick to note that MAOA deficiency "does not automatically lead to violence, or indeed any other kind of behavior" and that many people with MAOA deficiency do just fine (see Mann 1994, 1689). The point of such research, she stresses, is to discover what sort of support people with these problems need *in order* to be just fine (Mann 1994, 1689). Similarly, Hamer and Copeland claim that the "real reason to study the role of genes and biology in aggression is to understand what can be changed and what cannot, what works and what doesn't" (1998, 126–27). Once again, it is not that to be genetic is to be that which is unchangeable, but rather that which stands in need of (medical) intervention if it is to be changed successfully. "With many of these deficiencies," she states, "if you don't change the diet within the first year, it's too late" (Breakefield, quoted in Mann 1994, 1689).

There is, then, running through the history of research into the biological basis of crime, the continued hope that some simple, or at least tractable biological mechanism will be found to lie behind at least some sorts of criminality, one that will mark the biologically determined criminal and allow him to be identified and prevented from undertaking criminal actions *before* he has actually done so.[3] For the most part though, this tactic, while much discussed, is almost never tried, and has never met with the least success in actually reducing crime.[4] And yet, even if such claims never result in the sorts of actions that might be expected to reduce crime, the claims, as the next section will show, serve another purpose admirably, which is to direct attention away from the possible social and environmental causes of crime and toward attention to the nature of individual criminals.

The Individual as Criminal and Biology as Crime

Making the cause of violence out to be biological, and, further, genetic, is part of a program of making violence out to be the problem of the individual. If violence is caused by some biological problem internal to the individuals in question, then, it seems clear, society cannot be held to blame for its prevalence, nor can violent or criminal individuals make claims about links between their social situations and their behavior. This point is especially strong if it can be argued that a majority of the crime in a society can be shown to be linked to behavior that is in some way not part of the normal spectrum of behavior; that is, is in some way the result of a disease state. The articulation of the majority of violence and criminality as the result of brain disorder disassociates the society in question from the violence and crime. In chapter 7 a similar approach to understanding mood-affective disorders will be undertaken, where I will argue that the creation of depression as a genetic disease makes depression out to be the result of a biochemical disorder of the patient, and entirely disassociates it from the social system at large.

Depending on the claim in question, the excursions into hypothesized disorders in the criminal can be boldly blunt or quite subtle. Lombroso's biological criminals were marked, figuratively and literally, by their atavism, their disease state. The flurry of reports about and the excitement generated by the claim of a link between the XYY chromosomal anomaly and violent behavior was another of the rather bold hypotheses, as XYY men are indeed clearly marked by their chromosomal anomaly, as well as some physical problems. The only firm conclusions to come out of the vast research into XYY males is that some of them suffer minor intellectual deficits, including delayed language development, and on average may be slightly taller than the population mean (see Plomin et al. 1990, 144ff.). A small excess in the incarceration rate for XYY males remained even in carefully controlled studies, but this may have been an artifact of their slightly lower IQ, or perhaps their deviation from standard appearances, two things that make arrests more likely to end in convictions and jail time (see Patzer 1985, 60ff. and below) (See also Plomin et al. 1990, 146; Hamer and Copeland 1998, 108–10; Lewontin et al. 1984, 150; and Gould 1981, 143–45.) The single base-pair error that causes MAOA deficiency is said to be correlated with "aggressive outbursts" in most cases, and in individual cases with "arson, attempted rape, and exhibitionism" (Brunner et al. 1993). However, there is also a tendency toward "borderline mental retardation" (Brunner et al. 1993). What to make of this is unclear, since the XYY males' higher incarceration rate proved to be correlated with their reduced mental ability, but XYY males proved to be no more violent than the population at large—their higher incarceration rate was the result of mostly petty property crimes (see Plomin et al. 1990, 144ff.). It seems unlikely in the extreme that MAOA deficiency accounts for any great percentage of violent criminals (see Hamer and Copeland 1998, 116–20). Brunner et al. suggest, however, that the population rates of MAOA deficiency must be determined, and further study is needed on both the prevalence of *partial* (rather than complete) MAOA deficiency, and the relationship of partial MAOA deficiency and violence (Brunner et al. 1993). This seems to be a kind of suggestion that there might be some chance of social benefit accruing to this research in terms of the control of violence and violent crime

However, it seems certain that no class of criminals with any one clear biological stigma will account for any great percentage of criminal behavior, and likely that no large percentage of criminal behavior will come out of any *set* of distinct, clearly detectable biological problems. The move, then, is away from clear cases to more subtle forms of dysfunction. Obvious "criminal" traits as replaced by such things as "minor physical anomalies" (MPAs in the literature), minor variations in brain functioning such as "abnormal distributions" of hemisphere preference and EEGs (electroencephalograms), and by even vaguer hypothesized difficulties named by terms like minimal brain dysfunction (MBD, originally an acronym for "minimal brain damage").[5] While no one biological problem can account for any great percentage of criminals or crime, a host of disorders, ranging from clear metabolic disorders to merely hypothesized and undetectable "brain damage" can be imagined to account for those 4–6 percent of criminals who, it is said, commit over 50 percent of the crimes. This is said to be especially plausible with respect to violent crimes (see Mednick and Kandel, in Moffitt and Mednick, 1988).

Of course, with such vague criteria, there is next to no hope of "detecting" such "born" criminals before they commit crimes, and hence not much hope that detection and early intervention in this tiny minority of the population will really cut the crime rate in half as advertised. The problem is not simply that it is impossible to test for merely hypothesized brain disorders but also that most people who have even a cluster of the known traits correlated with criminal behavior will never be involved in a serious crime (see for example Gould 1981, 145, and Mann 1994, 1689).

Biology and Society: Violence and Social Action

Hamer and Copeland, in their discussion of violence and criminality, note that *neither* having "bad genes" *nor* being in a "bad environment" can adequately account for violent and troubled youth—nor for violent and troubled adults. They cite studies purporting to show that children without "problem" genes did fine regardless of environment, and even children *with* "problem" genes did fine as long as the environment they were raised in was "good." The problem was with those children who had both "bad genes" and "bad homes" (1998, 96–97). They claim that this showed that "genes made [some children] vulnerable" and represented a kind of "genetic sensitivity to the environment" (1998, 96–98). As additional evidence, they note that it is obvious that "social and environmental factors aren't enough to explain violence and crime" because if that "simple-minded view were true, then everybody born in the ghetto would be a criminal" (1998, 92).

This line of reasoning isn't new. Three researchers, Sweet, Mark, and Ervin, in what has become a famous and much quoted letter to *The Journal of the American Medical Association*, claimed that since only a small percentage of the "slum dwellers" took an active part in the inner-city riots of the late 1960s, and only a small percentage of those who took an active part "indulged in arson, sniping, and assault," conditions in those cities afflicted with urban riots could not be whole cause of them. Rather, they suggested, "brain dysfunction[s]" were the key to understanding why only some slum dwellers were unable "to resist the temptations of unrestrained violence" (Sweet et al., quoted in Lewontin et al. 1984, 169; see also Mark and Ervin 1970, 151–52). Mark and Ervin apply the same analysis to the police and National Guard members. They argue that relatively few "lost control" and killed people inappropriately, and hence that those that did may well have been suffering from brain dysfunctions; indeed, they may have been suffering from the same sorts of brain dysfunctions as the rioters (Mark and Ervin 1970, 150ff.). While Hamer and Copeland's approach is very up-to-date and genetic, the similarities between it and this older view are striking. Again, there is a small subset of the population being blamed for the vast majority of the crimes, and their biology is at the heart of it.

Both this new genetic model and the older view are centered on individual differences as being at the heart of things. The newer approach substitutes genes that make people susceptible to bad environments for "brain dysfunctions" but changes little else about the analysis. We might ask, though, a question that Mark and Ervin ignore entirely, and Hamer and Copeland treat as wholly nonproblematic. In the case of the riots Mark and Ervin refer to, what is it that makes participation in a violent protest a crime? What counts as *indulging* in arson, sniping, and assault, as opposed to *using* arson, sniping, and assault? Where is the line between an illegitimate protest, a violent revolution, and a civil war? There is, in other words, room to argue about whether the violence involved in those urban riots Sweet, Mark, and Ervin were referring to was justifiable.[6] While this is very controversial, that is exactly the point. What is going to *count* as crime is up to the society in question, at least in part. Where random acts of violence become terrorism, where terrorism becomes civil war, and where legitimate acts of war become attempts at genocide are not facts to be found outside of social systems. The claim that the most violent rioters were those suffering from brain disorders can only make sense within a system that sees the violence of rioters as a problem to be controlled, that sees the violence of rioters as dysfunctional and the rioters themselves as, therefore, brain-damaged. But as Patterson points out, sociobiological explanations of inner-city urban violence are relatively easy to come up with as well, explanations that make the sort of behavior condemned by Sweet, Mark, and Ervin out to be entirely rational (see Patterson 1995, 9). Whether high murder rates, high rates of violence, or frequent rioting are dysfunctional or not, though, the *assumption* that the individuals involved must be in some way abnormal is entirely unwarranted.

Hamer and Copeland are somewhat more sophisticated in their attempt to deal with this issue than were Sweet, Mark, and Ervin. They note that dealing with aggression and violence in society means "reducing poverty, improving education, eradicating slums, eliminating racism, and instilling discipline and respect for self and other" and that "aggression can play a useful role in society when it is channeled into appropriate forms of competition such as sports, games, the market economy, or at times of national peril, into defense" (1998, 127). Of course, one might think that "reducing poverty, improving education," and the like might be unobtainable goals for some populations at some times without recourse to aggressive violence or the threat of violence, which would be awkward for such a view. Kitcher, indeed, takes the desire to find genetic or biological links to violence and criminality as being explained by "a society that consistently and callously turns its back on programs that might aid the unfortunate" and would rather see problems as "hopeless" than as requiring the kind of money that the changes suggested by Hamer and Copeland would demand (Kitcher 1999, 24–5).

Hamer and Copeland, at least, understand a key point that much of the research and writing on the biological bases of violence and criminality miss entirely. The claim that the broad cross-cultural similarity in the patterns of criminal activity should lead us to think about biological causes is flawed in at least two ways. The most basic claim, that cross culturally a small proportion of the men are responsible for most of the crimes has not been shown in an adequate number of different societies to warrant treating it as a broad truism. But even if across different cultures it is true that a small minority of individuals commit the vast number of crimes, it is *not* the case that the general rates or types of crime are anything like the same in different cultures. Many of the heritability studies were carried out in Western Europe, where organized record keeping makes adoption studies easier to perform. While it is claimed that in both the United States and Denmark, for example, a small percentage of men commit most of the violent crimes, both the violent crime rates in these countries as well as the sorts of violent crimes committed are quite different (see for example Lester 1991 and Lester 1986). Even if we were to buy Harpending and Draper's sociobiological theory of the evolution of social and antisocial behavior (see above), the claim that the reason for different crime rates in, say, European and American cities is the result of population genetics should strain our credulity. In other words, I think it ought to seem unlikely that a different mix of the antisocial and the social genes in American and European cities is responsible for the different crime rates.

This is less a facetious objection than it might sound. Mark and Ervin argue that television violence cannot be a "principal" determinant of violence since Montreal and Boston have very different rates of violent crime but the same sort of TV. Since they argue that brain dysfunction may well be a principal determinant of violent behavior, I take it we are to believe that Montreal and Boston have very different rates of brain dysfunction (Mark and Ervin 1970, 150ff.).

Answering questions about why some inner cities in the United States, as opposed to cities in Western Europe, have such atrociously high murder rates quite likely has nothing to do with genetic variation, built-in biochemical disorders, or brain dysfunctions at all, and everything to do with a culture of violence and despair and easy access to high-powered firearms (see for example Hamer and Copeland 1998, 127; Kitcher 1999, 24; Lester 1991). Explaining the recent genocides in Rwanda and Burundi, for the most part carried out in a brutally personal way by individuals wielding nothing more sophisticated than blunt and vaguely edged weapons,[7] likely has nothing to do with any genes for violence or antisocial behavior, and nothing to do with reproductive strategies, however broadly we conceive of them. Rather, explaining these events demands reference to the brutal ethnic politics of radically unstable nations and the like—a politics the Western world helped create through its gross mismanagement and then abandonment of its African colonies. Research into the "genetics of violence" is unlikely to be of much help in explaining why some countries, but not others, undergo such terrible events.

However, to suggest that the explanation for differences in crime rates between countries or cities must be, at least in broad terms, environmental in origin is *not* to suggest that we have an environmental explanation available to us for *individual* differences. Part of what the biological research wanted to explain was, again, why only *some* people became violent criminals. Its failure to succeed at this task turned primarily on the conceptual limitations of research into human beings, or for that matter any other organisms in uncontrolled environments. But this doesn't mean that we have an answer for that question in terms of environment either. Thinking that the environment, and not the genetic or biochemical, is the right place to look in order to reduce the crime rate in the United States is not the same as thinking that the environment can answer questions about the individual differences. The latter question, I would argue, we have no good answer for, and no good way of getting an answer.

Genetic Import

While many researchers claim that there is evidence for a genetic link to violence and criminality, what to make of this purported link is unclear. Even if in any given society some small percentage of individuals with genetic disorders commit most of the crimes, the different rates of crime in different societies, as well as the different sorts of crimes committed, point toward a distinctly vital role for the environment—indeed, given the nature of crime, such evidence points especially toward the social environment. Given the huge difference in murder rates in major cities in Western Europe and those in the United States, it might seem that concentrating on the genetic is, contra Moffitt and Mendick, the wrong way to think about reducing crime. Even if every hypothesized congenital criminal in the United States were "cured" or locked away before doing any harm, the crime rate would still be well above that of many other advanced Western societies, all of whose hypothesized congenital criminals would remain free. This is because, obviously, the crime rates in such different societies differ by well over the 50 percent of crime said to be accountable for by the small number of hypothesized congenital criminals.

The focus on the genetic and biological causes of crime, then, is not wrong because we can know that there are none. Rather, it is wrong because we know that the largest differences in the rates of crime between different societies are the result of different environments, especially different social environments and modes of social organization. It is unlikely in the extreme that any of the differences in the rates of crime, including violent crime, between societies could possibly be accounted for by anything like different genetic distributions between the societies in question. The focus on the genetic becomes a way of not focusing on the role of the environment. It may be possible to intervene medically, as it may well be the case that within this environment there are discoverable links between biology and crime. But even if such a link exists, it will be dependent on the environment, and intervening at the level of the individual will be only one possible way of intervening. In the case of violence and criminality, it seems clear, this would not be anything like the best way. Rather than attempting to understand why one inner-city youth adopts a life of crime and violence while another does not, we perhaps ought to concentrate our limited resources on understanding why so many more violent crimes per capita occur in the United States than in many other Western nations.

CHAPTER 6
GAY GENES AND THE REIFICATION OF HOMOSEXUALITY

Why Study Sexual Orientation?

Contemporary studies of the heritability and genetics of homosexuality usually explicitly state that it is not part of their goal to enable changes to be made; this contrasts sharply with many other human genetic studies, such as those into the genetic etiologies of various physical diseases, mental disorders, or antisocial behaviors.[1] In the case of physical diseases, mental diseases, and (to a lesser extent) antisocial behaviors, the standard story is that it is explanation and prediction with an eye toward intervention that makes them worth doing. Given this sort of raison d'être in the case of most studies, then, the purpose of studies on the heritability and genetics of homosexuality is always somewhat in doubt, as intervention, at least, is generally considered an unacceptable goal, and prediction is often thought to be too closely linked to intervention at the level of, for example, prenatal screening and abortion, for it to be an acceptable goal.[2] In one version of the story, the research is supposed to be of interest simply because of the intrinsic interest in the subject (see Horgan 1993; Hamer and Copeland 1994, 19–20). In another version of the story, the hope is that showing that homosexuality is innate and genetically influenced, or at least biological, will tend to increase tolerance of homosexuals (see Horgan 1993, quoting Simon LeVay; Murphy 1997, 56; but see also Hamer and Copeland 1994, 19–20).

Neither of these responses is particularly satisfying, however, and both have at least hints of a particularly dangerous disingenuity about them.

The expectation that finding some partial biological "causes" of homosexuality would have any effect on social tolerance seems, for example, startlingly naive.[3] Certainly, there is no evidence for any biological correlates to homosexuality that is as certain as is the evidence that, in this culture, sexual orientation is not for the most part anything like a matter of "choice," and is pretty much impossible to change (at least deliberately).[4]

But the very attempt to show that homosexuality is biologically "caused" and hence should be "tolerated" buys too much into a medical model of homosexuality, and de facto makes it out to be an abnormal state. Indeed, this should be thought of in direct opposition to, for example, increasing social tolerance of people suffering from Tourette's syndrome by showing it to have a primarily biological, and perhaps a genetic, etiology. Most people would readily agree that sufferers from Tourette's syndrome, at least its severe forms, act in ways that are far outside the normal variation in behavior, and further in ways that are generally regarded as socially unacceptable. The question then becomes how to treat these behavioral aberrations (see Mann 1994). However, the increase in "social toleration" that follows an understanding of the etiology of Tourette's syndrome does *not* take the form of making the behaviors socially acceptable; rather it takes the form of recognizing that the sufferers cannot help but engage in unacceptable behavior. This is, I take it, *not* the sort of "social toleration" most homosexuals, nor for that matter most people who support the rights of homosexuals, would approve of. And it is by this parallel with Tourette's that I believe it can be most easily seen that people who suspect that social tolerance of homosexuality will follow from the discovery of biological causes are dealing with a radically medicalized model of homosexuality. If an effective treatment for Tourette's were developed we would *expect* suffers to avail themselves of it, and therefore to stop shouting obscenities and touching people and things in socially inappropriate ways. If one thinks that homosexuality, in this culture, is simply part of the normal range of behaviors, the implications of expecting "social tolerance" to be increased because of a medicalization of the condition are very deeply disturbing.[5]

On the other hand, why homosexuality should be of sufficient intrinsic interest to warrant studying as a possible genetically influenced trait remains an open question. After all, the Minnesota Twin Study suggests a high genetic component to "job satisfaction" (Arvey et al. 1994) and yet there has been no suggestion that a study aimed at finding the relevant genes would even be potentially interesting or useful. Still less has there been any suggestion that further research into the "remarkable" and "bewitching" parallels that Bouchard claimed to find between reunited twins in this study might be useful, and less still that undertaking a linkage and direct sequence study of those odd traits would prove interesting and worth funding; no one is prepared to pay to try to find genes associated with idiosyncratic toilet-flushing habits, wearing shirts with epaulets, or the other "bewitching" parallels (see Horgan 1993). Murphy notes that ceteris paribus "there probably are reasons why some people systematically prefer strawberry to butterscotch flavorings, or vanilla to chocolate" (1997, 47), but that these have so far not been the subject of much scientific investigation—the possible genetic etiology of preferring vanilla has been the subject of neither heritability studies nor molecular searches.

A plausible account of this difference follows from the common expectation, in this culture, that a person's sexuality is, in Halperin's formulation, somehow a "constitutive feature of his or her personality"; that is, that in this culture a person's sexuality makes them a "type" of person, a homosexual or heterosexual (Halperin 1990, 27). We do not, in other words, expect a person's score on some job satisfaction index, or preference for ice-cream flavors, to tell us anything particularly interesting about the sort of person they are; but for us, sexuality, and specifically sexual orientation, is one of the ways in which we categorize individuals; we do expect that *these* categories, unlike flavor preferences, will tell us interesting things about the world. Part of the appeal of research into sexuality, then, may well be the expectation that people's sexuality will be linked up with other potentially deep and interesting traits in a way that their score on a job satisfaction index or their ice-cream preferences will not.[6]

But on one view of sexuality, it is not *intrinsically* linked to other interesting and deep traits at all. Halperin and Foucault, for example, argue that the categories of homosexuality and heterosexuality were created, and created rather recently. Further, they argue that the creation of homosexuality as a category of behavior went hand in hand with the creation of homosexuality as defining a kind of person, rather than simply being a collection of different types of behaviors that were a matter of personal preference or taste. Dupré notes that "given the arbitrariness of the decision to treat homosexuals and heterosexuals as *kinds* of people in the first place" the search for biological and genetic differences between them "may be no more firmly grounded than the search for the typical characteristics and genetic peculiarities of stamp collectors or aficionados of crossword puzzles" (Dupré 1993, 253, emphasis in original).

Insofar as any such correlates are found, whether for homo- or heterosexuality or for stamp collecting, there is the risk of creating, or at least reinforcing, the trait *as* a type; that is, of legitimating its use as a way of organizing the world. Indeed, we might say that the very search for such correlates implies the importance of the search—the search itself presupposes at the very least the *coherence* of there being some kinds of biological correlates or others, and reveals assumptions about what sorts of traits stand in need of biological explanations. Finding such correlates implies the importance, or at least the naturalness, of the type. But if with, for example, Appiah, one wonders about the wisdom of the cultural assumption that any personal traits are going to be correlated with other deep and interesting traits, any research that directly or indirectly makes this sort of typing seem more natural is going to seem very suspect indeed (see Appiah 1994). (More on this below.)

In this chapter, I will explore the way that even research that is well done from a *technical* point of view can carry with important social dangers and be misleading both scientifically and socially. The problems, I will argue, with, for example, Hamer's work in genetic linkage studies on male homosexuality have nothing to do with failures in scientific methodology. Rather, the difficulties with properly interpreting the results of Hamer's research stem almost entirely from the conceptual difficulties in dealing with complex and socially mediated human behaviors. Indeed, I will argue that the context dependence of genetic associations is adequate to explain the consistent failure of other research teams to replicate the results of Hamer's studies. Hamer's work, like so many studies on human genetics, comes up against a dilemma: insofar as it is not overinterpreted or misinterpreted, it is able to show little or nothing; that is, it provides no basis for prediction, explanation, or control in the world, and insofar as it seems to hint that it might provide such a basis, it risks gross and dangerous over- and misinterpretation.

The Heritability and Genetics of Homosexuality

Some studies of sexual orientation seem to imply that the broad-sense heritability of sexual orientation is somewhere in the .3–.7 range (see Hamer and Copeland 1994, 29–30). However, even these vague numbers should be interpreted cautiously, given the small number of studies and the lack of methodological variation—there have been, for example, no full adoption studies that explored sexual orientation. At this time, it is also unclear how distinct the etiologies of male and female homosexuals are. In most studies, however, brothers of both male and female homosexuals were more likely to be homosexual than males without homosexual siblings; similarly, sisters of both male and female homosexuals were more likely to be homosexual themselves then females without homosexual siblings (see Bailey and Bell 1993, especially the summary of studies, 317). This is sometimes thought to point toward at least a hint of a partial similarity in causal history. Pattatucci and Hamer argue that the etiology of female sexual orientation is probably at least partially distinct from that of male sexual orientation (see Pattatucci and Hamer 1995, 408), and Hamer and Copeland argue that they are probably "fundamentally distinct" (1998, 191–92). It should also be noted that studies of identical twins regularly generate concordance rates for homosexuality in the .5 range, and usually on the low side of that range, which makes the highest estimates of broad-sense heritability seem rather far-fetched (see Horgan 1993).

Hamer's work in finding a linkage between a marker on the X chromosome and a gene believed to influence sexual orientation had the advantage of sidestepping many issues in heritability studies. Indeed, his methodology, working on "concordant" brothers, sidestepped many of the difficulties with most linkage studies. Hamer concentrated on gay brothers, and used only the shared-trait sib-pair method to look for linkage.[7] The idea behind this method is elegantly simple. A pair of siblings who share a phenotypic trait, in this case homosexuality, will share some heterogeneous genetic marker more often than could be expected on average if that marker is linked to a gene that is positively correlated with the phenotypic trait in question.[8] Since Hamer had already determined that the gene he was looking for a linkage with was somewhere on the X chromosome, he had merely to test pairs of gay brothers and see if they'd inherited the same marker from their mother; that is, to see if they had gotten the same bit of the same X chromosome from her. If gay brothers shared the same marker, and hence shared a piece of their mother's X chromosome, more often than they would be expected to by chance, that piece was implicated as being correlated with homosexuality. Famously, Hamer found a marker (around Xq28) highly correlated with male homosexuality in the population he studied. (Hamer et al., 1993).[9]

Besides having produced a clever research design, Hamer displays a striking humility with respect to what his research actually shows. He notes that his work does not "address the role of the Xq28 locus in the population at large or even among all gay men" (Hamer and Copeland 1994, 144–45). Among the questions that "remain to be answered" Hamer lists:

> What fraction of all gay men carry an Xq28-linked allele that influenced their sexual orientation? What is the frequency of this allele among heterosexual men? How many different alleles are present at Xq28, and what is the effect of each? What other genes and nongenetic factors influence sexual orientation, and what role does each play? (Hamer 1994, 145)

Hamer further notes that even answering such questions within a "particular population, say residents of Washington, D.C.," would still not permit any assumptions about the application of these answers to "other populations" and notes that the social environment might well influence the expression of any genes found (Hamer and Copland 1994, 145). This would seem to suggest that the very recent failure of a study in Canada to confirm a linkage at Xq28 (Rice et al. 1999) is not entirely surprising. Finally, Hamer notes that despite the strength of the linkage, finding the gene itself, let alone explicating the biochemical or causal pathway by which it works, will certainly prove very difficult, and may be impossible with current technology and methods (Hamer and Copland 1994, 147–48).[10]

Perhaps most interesting is Hamer's own discomfort with his work. His and his colleagues' first paper in *Science* ended not with an ordinary conclusion or notes for future work, but with a comment on the moral implications of the work. The final paragraph reads (in full):

> Our work represents an early application of molecular linkage methods to a normal variation in human behavior. As the human genome project proceeds, it is likely that many such correlations will be discovered. We believe that it would be fundamentally unethical to use such information to try to assess or alter a person's current or future sexual orientation, either heterosexual or homosexual, or other normal attributes of human behavior. Rather, scientists, educators, policy-makers, and the public should work together to ensure that such research is used to benefit all members of society. (Hamer et al. 1993)

Their stress on treating homosexuality as representing part of the normal variation in human sexuality is itself revealing, because of course, for most of this century it has not been treated as "normal" at all (see for example Halperin 1990), and even today such a claim remains contentious.

Again, if such claims *weren't* contentious, no claims about the biology of homosexuality could even be *relevant* to the dominant view of homosexuality and the hope of, for instance, increasing social tolerance. *Normal* variations in human behavior, I take it, do not stand in need of a biological basis to be acceptable. That is, no one tries to elucidate biological bases for those things that we take to be part of the normal range of behavior in our society, and insofar as many behaviors within the normal range of behavior in our society have some biological basis or other, this isn't considered the *reason* that they are acceptable. Even if someone did find a genetic marker, or even a gene, associated with a preference for vanilla over chocolate *ceteris paribus* (to follow Murphy's example, see above), that wouldn't be the *reason* that preferring one to the other was acceptable. (See above on the comparison to the social acceptance of those socially *unacceptable* behaviors associated with Tourette's syndrome.)

But it is the final sentence of Hamer's conclusion that is perhaps most interesting, because given the list of unanswered questions, the incomplete penetrance of the genetic, especially in these sorts of complex behaviors, and the obvious and admitted massive influence of the environment, it is completely unclear what benefit "such research" *could* have to *any* members of society. This question is especially troubling given Hamer's insistence that such research should not be used for prediction or control of the traits in question. The research, then, yields results that are at best minimally explanatory in some very local situations, and that the researchers claim cannot and should not be used for prediction or control of the world—*cannot* because the research doesn't support the sorts of results that would be necessary for prediction and control, and *should not* because in any event prediction and control would be morally repugnant.

At this point, the danger of such research must be obvious. Interpreted as strictly as Hamer seems to wish, at least when he is writing or speaking carefully and precisely, it shows nothing outside of a very specific linkage associated with a trait in very specific circumstances, within a very small population in a rather narrow environment. The research, if we are to believe Hamer, presupposes the normality of the trait in question and cannot be considered more than a methodological first step toward beginning to explicate a small piece of a causal pathway.[11] But given a notion of sexuality that makes it out to be central to who and what we are, the creation of a research project designed to find differences between heterosexuals and homosexuals cannot help but be fit into a social system that makes sexuality out to be something real and deeply linked to who and what we are. Hamer's work, for all its careful methodology, is, as Halperin puts it, just the sort of research that "is designed to confirm current categories of analysis rather than to call those very categories into question" (Halperin 1990, 50), and it is in at least in part because it does that so well, and so unself-consciously, that it represents so great a danger.

The Contingency of Sexuality

Hamer's work contained within it an explicit definition of homosexuality; individuals only counted as homosexual if they scored either 5 or 6 on the Kinsey scale of self-identification, attraction, fantasy, and behavior (see Hamer et al. 1993). The Kinsey scale breaks various aspects of sexual orientation down into seven discrete categories, with 0 being "exclusively heterosexual," 6 being "exclusively homosexual," and 3 being "fully bisexual." Generally, people are scored by asking them questions like the following one (on attraction), taken from Hamer's research:

> ... zero stands for exclusively attracted to females and six stands for exclusively attracted to males. Suppose you walk into a party, you notice various people, and you think to yourself, "That one might be interesting to go to bed with." What sex would that person be? (Hamer and Copeland 1994, 59)

In the primarily white and middle-class men in the Washington, D.C., area that Hamer studied, most scored either 0 or 1, or 5 or 6, on the four Kinsey scales that Hamer checked (self-identification, attraction, fantasy, and behavior). Very few of the men recorded scores in the 2–4 range. This, Hamer claimed, put most men either firmly in the class of heterosexuals or that of homosexuals (see Hamer and Copeland 1994, 67; and Hamer et al. 1993). (Interestingly, this does not seem to be the case in the population of women Pattatucci and Hamer studied. See below for discussion.)

Cross-cultural studies of male homosexuality, however, paint a somewhat different picture. While in Hamer's study relatively few self-identified heterosexual men regularly engaged in homosexual intercourse or scored above a 1 on the attraction index, Whitam and Mathy point out that in, for instance, Guatemala the situation is rather different, with some studies showing that some "eighty percent of heterosexual males regularly have secondary homosexual contact" (1986, 134), and Halperin makes a similar point about the sexual practices and sensibilities of some current Mediterranean cultures (1990, 61).

Halperin wonders about the status of genetic or biological "causes" of homosexuality with respect to various different cultural traditions. If, he argues, we hypothesize a cross-culturally genetic or biological cause, what are we to say of cultures where the homosexual/heterosexual distinction is less clear than in ours? He asks us to consider a New Guinea tribesman

> who from ages eight to fifteen has been orally inseminated on a daily basis by older youths and who, after years of orally inseminating his juniors, will be married to an adult woman and have children of his own. ... According to our hypothesis, science will now be able to reveal definitely whether he is or is not gay. Neither alternative, though, is going to be very satisfactory. For, according to one possibility, the tribesman isn't *really* gay—he just spends half his life having oral sex with other males ... according to the only other possibility, the tribesman really *is* gay, but then how shall we explain why he shows no

erotic interest in males outside of initiatory contexts or why he does not hesitate to marry and not experience any sexual difficulty in his adult relations with women? (Halperin 1990, 46, 48; emphasis in original)

Of course, one perfectly reasonable thing to say is that genes express themselves differently in different environments, and a gene that is correlated with male homosexuality in, for example, some upper-middle-class white men in the Washington, D.C., area is not necessarily likely to be so correlated in other environments or populations.

In a sense, of course, such a response misses at least part of the point of Halperin's example. It is not just that whatever genetic and environmental correlates to homosexuality happen to exist in this culture may not be correlated with homosexuality in other cultures. Rather, other cultures may lack the concept of homosexuality, lack "homosexuality" and "heterosexuality" as categories that work to define sorts of people. Where the object of sexual attraction is not considered of interest, or at least not considered the sort of thing that defines a person, any biological or genetic correlates to such a choice might be beside the point. Further, as will be discussed in more detail below, such correlations may well not exist in those cultures that organize their sexual lives differently.

There are at least two descriptions of sexual behavior within cultures with different ways of organizing sexuality that are relevant to this issue. In one description, whatever way the culture organizes sexuality, people still act in ways that form recognizable patterns from the standpoint of sexual orientation. If even in cultures that don't use sexual orientation as their primary organizational axis for sexuality, people's behavior still fell along lines that made sense of those categories, the argument about the contingency of the categories would lose much of its bite. If whatever the social organization of sexuality was, individuals organized their own sexual lives (at least primarily) around sexual orientation, this would be an interesting observation. We might even suppose that they did so unconsciously, such that the gender of the object of desire would never be mentioned or thought of as significant, but most individuals would reveal a strong preference for a particular gender in their sexual behavior, whatever the categories in use within society were.

Again, though, this doesn't seem to be the case; sexual behavior is not consistent cross-culturally (see above). The way in which a culture organizes and interprets sexuality does seem to influence the individual behavior of its members, often in important ways. Indeed, a current argument is about how to interpret the differences in male and female sexuality within this culture.

Recall again that for men in the populations studied, Hamer argued that most were either firmly in the class of heterosexuals or homosexuals, based on their scoring either mostly 0 or 1, or mostly 5 or 6, on the four Kinsey scales of self-identification, attraction, fantasy, and behavior, with very few recording scores in the 2–4 range for any of these scales (see Hamer et al. 1993). However, for the women Pattatucci and Hamer studied, stable bisexuality, both in terms of self-identification and behavior, was relatively common, and certainly much more common than it had been for men. Further, for women the results of Kinsey designations based on self-identification were not as predictive of those results based on the designators of romantic/sexual attraction, romantic/sexual fantasy, or sexual behavior as they were for men. That is, far more women who were, say, Kinsey 1s in terms of self-identification admitted to having been romantically/sexually attracted to other women, and far more women who were Kinsey 5s or 6s admitted having been romantically/sexually attracted to men, than did men with those self-identified Kinsey ratings admit to being attracted to other men or women, respectively (Pattatucci and Hamer 1995, esp. 410–12).

In interpreting these striking differences, Hamer, for example, is willing to consider them as either emerging out of the different sexual environments men and women are born into in this culture, or to interpret them as deeply biological, and claims to simply be awaiting some evidence one way or the other (Hamer 1995,). The environmental interpretation is of obvious interest here, especially given the differences in the way same-sex sexual contact and admitted attraction among heterosexual men to men is treated in, for example, the United States versus, for example, in certain Latin America and Mediterranean cultures (see Carrier 1976; Whitam and Mathy 1986; Halperin 1990). Faderman's work on same-sex relationships among women in relatively recent (sixteenth-to-eighteenth-century) Western history makes a similar point: the availability of the category "romantic friendship" to describe these relationships and the lack of stigma attached to this category created the conditions for the expression of desires that might otherwise never have existed, let alone been expressed (Faderman 1981, 1994). In short, the existence, or lack thereof, of categories to organize various forms of sexual expression *does* seem to influence human behavior, not just descriptions of behavior.

It is for this reason that Foucault's approach to ancient Greek sexual behavior is so interesting. In Foucault's interpretation, ancient Greek men were not "bisexual"; as they failed to recognize any principled difference between sexual attraction to boys and women, their "sexuality" (insofar as this term could even be said to apply—see below) was not "dual, ambivalent" but rather "was simply the appetite that nature had implanted in man's heart for 'beautiful' human beings" (Foucault 1985, 188). Halperin, with Foucault, argues that there is no evidence that the Greeks had any category like our "homosexual," a category that captured all and only people attracted to members of the same sex (see for example Halperin 1990, 19–22). Part of what this meant was that for the ancient Greeks, the man who hires a male prostitute was *not* in any category similar to that of the male prostitute he hires (Halperin 1990, 96–97; see also Foucault 1985, 46–47).

Indeed, Halperin claims that sexuality did not exist per se for the ancient Greeks; rather, he argues, their relationship to what we would term sexuality should be thought of "as a more generalized ethos of penetration and domination" (1990 34, 36). As "the classical Athenians . . . tended *both* to construct social and sexual roles hierarchically *and* to collapse the distinctions between them, associating sexual penetration and phallic pleasure alike with social domination" the role one took in sex vis-à–vis one's role with respect to penetration was linked to one's social status (Halperin 1990, 97; emphasis in original). It was, that is, the active/passive distinction that was key, and adult Athenian male citizens could lose their citizenship if they were found to have, as adults, permitted themselves to be put into positions where they would be in the passive sexual role, such as if they were found to have prostituted themselves (Halperin 1990, 96–97; see also Laqueur 1990, 52–53). Sex between political equals was, then, simply impossible, and for this reason sex in "classical Athens" should, Halperin argued, be thought of as "a deeply polarizing experience," one that "divides, classifies, and distributes its participants into distinct and radically opposed categories" (1990, 30). There was, though, no problem with sex between male citizens and women, slaves, foreigners,[12] or statutory minors, as long as it was the male citizen who took the active role in intercourse. In each case, the male citizen, taking the active role, is gendered as male within an "ethos of phallic penetration and domination," and the "passive" participant is gendered as female; that is, as lacking a phallus and thus being in the position of that which is penetrated (Halperin 1990, 34–35). The male who penetrates was, then, engaged in a completely different sort of activity from the male who permitted himself to be penetrated, and belonged to an entirely different category of person.[13]

Whether there existed individuals in ancient Athens who were primarily attracted to members of the same gender, despite the lack of a way of categorizing that desire, remains something of an open question, and one not easily answered by the historical information available. However, even if such people did exist, it seems clear that their way of interpreting and acting on those desires would be very different from those of a contemporary homosexual; specifically, it seems very likely that they would interpret their desires through the prism of a "sexuality" focused on power relationships. In any event, it seems at least somewhat likely that many ancient Athenian males participated in and enjoyed a range of sexual behaviors that in most parts of the contemporary culture of the United States would be viewed as deeply problematic; of course, ancient Athenians would no doubt find contemporary sexual practices in the United States deeply problematic as well.

In contemporary Western cultures, and especially in the United States, Faderman points out that "both heterosexual and homosexual social life demand commitment to the category" (1994, 15). The result of this demand of commitment to the categories is that "the identities heterosexual and homosexual thus become entrenched" (1994, 15). Any form of sexuality that denies that sexual orientation is the right divide, or even attempts to position itself outside that divide, will therefore seem especially deviant and problematic. Organization along the axis of sexual orientation, then, effectively prevents the expression, and possibly the formation, of any sexual desires that do not take as fundamental sexual orientation as the primary way of categorization (1994, 15).

Constructions and Scripting

The above analysis suggests both that the concepts that apply to what we would call "sexuality" are not stable cross-culturally, and that those categories deeply affect who we are and how we deal with the world. That is, who we find attractive, how we think of the relationships between sex and the political world, and the like are deeply influenced by the categories of thought our cultures make available to us. Sexuality on this view is, at least in large part, constructed, socially constituted, and contingent. While the notion of traits being "social constructions" has, unfortunately, become rather a loaded issue, I merely mean something like the following by this way of phrasing the issue: Societies have and do organize sexuality in different ways and along different axes. Individuals' ways of conceiving of themselves in sexual terms follow at least in part from the ways in which their societies organize sexuality. Not only does one's self-description emerge in part out of the way society organizes sexual expression, but also such things as who one finds attractive and who one actually has sex with will vary based in part on the way one's culture organizes sexuality. The last section argued that the main axis along which contemporary Western society organizes sexuality—sexual orientation—is contingent in at least several ways. Some societies don't organize or haven't organized sexuality in that way, and people in those societies behave differently with respect to same-sex sexual relationships, and indeed, sexual relationships in general, than do people in the United States and some other contemporary Western societies. Further, that American society currently organizes sexuality along the lines of sexual orientation is no evidence for such a mode of organization's having a long history in Western culture, nor does it suggest that such a way of organizing sexuality is likely to be a permanent feature of even the United States's society. I believe that to take this as implying that sexuality is a social construction and contingent is accurate, as far it goes (see also Stein 1998).

But even if sexuality is a construct in this way, our concepts of homosexuality and heterosexuality are not, as Halperin points out, merely "categories of thought"; they are also, for example, "categories of erotic response" and as such "describe zones of freedom, pleasure, and erotic excitement" (Halperin 1990, 53). Our categories of sexuality make up a large part of our concepts of the self, and as such they are not categories one could, even in principle, "think oneself out of" (1990, 53).

This, though, makes the thesis that our sexuality is constructed, socially constituted, and contingent somewhat counterintuitive (perhaps, Halperin suggests, necessarily so), as "our intuitions about the world and about ourselves are no doubt constituted at the same time as our sexuality itself" (1990, 44). Despite Halperin's claim that "gay sub-cultures provide abundant evidence for the vast plurality of possible sexual styles" such that it must be obvious "that "sexuality" is not the sort of thing that comes in only two kinds (i.e., 'hetero-' and 'homo-')," he yet admits that "I don't think there's any way that I, or anyone else who grew up in bourgeois America when I did, could ever believe in what I've been saying with the same degree of conviction with which I believe, despite everything I've said, in the categories of heterosexuality and homosexuality" (1990, 44, 53). Halperin's response to being asked if the social construction and contingency of the categories hetero- and homosexual doesn't "contradict what many people claim to 'know' about themselves" seems to be that insofar as it does, the only honest intellectual position is to admit that while we might not be able to believe in the contingency and construction of the categories with the same conviction we are forced to believe in the categories themselves, yet we "can affirm" their contingency and construction "with solid intellectual conviction" (1990, 44, 53).

Given this, how are we to interpret research like Hamer's? His research takes categories that are culturally contingent, but, as suggested above, are something we may feel stuck with, as a proper starting point for a causal analysis. That is to say, insofar as we take research into the causal pathways of homosexuality—or, for that matter, heterosexuality—as problematic, how do we fit this problematization into a recognition that homosexuality and heterosexuality really are the major categories we use, in this culture, for defining and dealing with our own and other people's sexuality? Of course, one obvious form of problematization was suggested above. Insofar as our culture is living,[14] there is the opportunity for its constructs to change with it, to change as it changes. When Halperin suggests that gay subcultures today actually display the inadequacy of the hetero/homo dichotomy, part of what he is suggesting is that different sorts of sexualities, different ways of organizing the sexual world, are becoming available, or at the very least might become available (1990, 44). We can learn, he suggests, "how idiosyncratic and various, how unsystematic sexuality is" and how many different classification schemes are available (1990, 44). When Halperin asks, somewhat rhetorically, "is a gay woman into S/M more like a gay woman who is not or a straight woman who is?" it seems that at least one of the answers we might give is that there is no necessary fact of the matter, that whatever answer we give is culturally mediated (1990, 44).[15]

Again, though, this doesn't change the fact that in this culture, homo- and heterosexuality are categories used to type people much more readily than, for example, specifically what sexual activities one enjoys. As Hamer notes, "[m]ost people . . . would say they have a good idea who is gay and who is straight in their own families" and that "measuring sexual orientation is something we do informally all the time" (Hamer and Copeland 1994, 53). The same cannot be said of what specific sorts of sexual practices people engage in; most of us, I take it, have little or no idea about our different family members' relative fondness for, for example, oral-genital intercourse or anal stimulation. But of course, this doesn't make those categories we use to type people any deeper or more real in a metaphysical way than those categories that we don't so use (see for example Dupré 1993). Again, recall that for at least some of the ancient Greeks, it was a (male) citizen's desire to be in the passive homosexual role, to be penetrated, that was considered unnatural and stood in desperate need of explanation (see Laqueur 1990, 44). In that culture, the specific sexual activities one enjoyed had a social and political meaning, and were *in fact* a way of typing people, in the way that the *object* of sexual interest was not.

If, for the ancient Greeks, what specific sexual activities one enjoyed was not an issue about personal tastes, but, being a matter of deep social consequence involving domination, rather carried with it certain social roles and expectations, so too for our culture is one's sexual orientation not considered a matter of personal taste, but rather carries with it a set of expectations about other aspects of one's life. The reason "many people would claim to be able to point out at least some of the . . . gay . . . men and women passing by" (Hamer and Copeland 1994, 53) clearly has nothing to do with their being able to get a historical fix on the relative frequency of the sexes/genders of the sexual partners of those people passing by. Rather it has to do with the way one's sexuality is assumed to be, and in fact often is, tied into a nest of other traits, traits that can then be read as revealing one's sexuality.

To some extent, of course, our ability to do this isn't a myth at all. Sexuality in this culture often does come with a package of traits. Such very preliminary results on the ability of both men and women to success-fully classify straight and openly gay speakers of American English based on voice alone are very suggestive in the context (see Gaudio 1994), as is the phenomena of "gaydar," the claimed ability of homosexuals to identify other homosexuals in contexts where sexual orientation isn't transparent. However robust a phenomena this is, and some very bold claims are often made surrounding it, the existence of the term and widespread belief in its efficacy are, I take it, themselves evidence that sexuality is assumed to be linked to other traits in this culture. (see for example "Boy George, I Think He's Got It," box, 63).

One way to cash out this nest of traits is, with Appiah, to note that cer-tain ways of categorizing people result in "collective identities" that come with "loose norms or models" of "modes of behavior" that "play a role in shaping the life plans of those make these collective identities central to their individual identities" (1994, 159). We can speak, Appiah claims, of these identities coming with "what we might call scripts: narratives that people can use in shaping their life plans and telling their life stories" (1994, 160). Faderman is making a similar point when she notes that the "existence of the categories homosexual and heterosexual freezes one in an entire identity from which it is not easy to move, even if circumstances should warrant it, because an entire social life is built around that identity" (Faderman 1994, 17). Certainly, in our culture being a "homosexual" puts one in such a category in a way that one's specific tastes in sexual activities do not. That is, I take it that being someone who is rather more fond of penile-anal than penile-vaginal intercourse does not come with a script in this culture, and again, it is something we would consider an irrelevant fea-ture of the sexual lives of our family members and friends, unlike their relationship vis-à–vis the hetero- and homosexuality divide. Further, I think it is interesting to note the "unnatural" feel of those categories to us.

Without additional reference to the gender and relative position of the participants—facts that would de facto constitute them in relationship to our concepts of sexuality and sexual orientation—these categories simply don't speak to us at all. That is, given the ways of organizing sexuality we have in contemporary society, "being more fond of penile-anal than penile-vaginal intercourse" doesn't seem to us to be a category at all. In part, I take it, this is because it seems to be a very different thing to say this of, for example, homosexual men, heterosexual men, and heterosexual women.

While who gets to write the life-scripts ends up mattering a great deal, such scripts will always be somewhat limiting, both in terms of what one can do as well as what one can think. As Appiah points out, part of what one is doing when one attempts to "construct a series of positive gay life-scripts" in response to a generally homophobic community is demanding that one not be "treated with equal dignity *despite* being homosexual" (emphasis added) but rather that one be "respected as a homosexual" (1994, 162). Appiah observes that this may be a "historically, strategically necessary" move, and I think he is certainly right to prefer "the world of gay liberation" to "the world of the closet"; however, he is also quite correct in noting that the life-script of the homosexual, whether written by the homophobic culture at large or by the homosexual community itself, carries with it certain dangers as well (1994, 162–63). Any life-script is going to be limiting, even if it is a "positive" one. Moreover, it is again unclear if any account can be "so positive as to be proof against hostile appropriation and transformation" (Halperin 1990, 52).

In wanting "other options" to the closet or gay liberation, in wanting people to be able to "treat . . . their sexual body as [a] personal dimension . . . of the self," Appiah is suggesting that treating sexuality and sexual orientation as simply a matter of personal taste should be a real option (1994, 162–63). Appiah argues that our sexuality ought to be something that doesn't come with a script, or at least as something that is "not too tightly scripted" and which we shouldn't have to "organize [our] life around" (1994, 163). Similarly, Halperin thinks that we "must acknowledge that "sexuality" is a cultural production no less than are table manners, health clubs, and abstract expressionism, and we must struggle to discern in what we currently regard as our most precious, unique, original, and spontaneous impulses the traces of a previously rehearsed and socially encoded ideological script" (1990, 40). Through this, Halperin thinks, we can come "to admit that what seem to be our most inward, authentic, and private experiences are actually . . . "shared, unnecessary and political'" (1990, 40, quoting Adrienne Rich). Recognizing this will be related,

Halperin suggests, to the "endless undertaking" of "distinguishing freedom from constraint in love, of learning to trace the shifting and uncertain boundaries between the self and the world" (1990, 40). Faderman makes a similar point about the positive possibilities inherent in the construction of human sexuality with less emphasis on categories when she notes that "without the power and tyranny of the categories, human sexuality and affectionality could easily be undifferentiated" from the standpoint of sexual orientation (1994, 15).

One way of conceiving of the issue, then, is not as primarily about whether society should find new ways of organizing sexuality along grand axes, but whether such forms of organization, which are themselves deeply limiting, can be avoided entirely.

Biology and Scripts

Part of the problem with, for example, Hamer's work, is just that it seems to make homosexuality out to be a thing that can—and, by implication at least, should—be studied, and hence reinforces the idea that there is something important and distinctive about the contemporary categories of sexuality this culture uses. When Hamer says that the expression of whatever gene it is that is linked to Xq28 and correlated with homosexuality in white males in the Washington, D.C., area might vary in different environments, he hides the complete irrelevance of the category "homosexual" to many environments in which the gene might find itself.

But perhaps it would be better to say that it is the environment of the person who in our culture *would be* carrying such a gene that makes the gene irrelevant. That is to say, the difficulty with how to treat a gene that supposedly codes for homosexuality in, say, middle-aged white males in Washington, D.C., in a culture where "homosexuality" not only comes without a script but also does not exist as a way of classifying people, should strike us as a very deep problem indeed. In a culture whose concepts of sexuality and behavioral practices do not map onto ours, what role could a gene that codes for homosexuality in our culture play? This is of course rather closely related to the more general question of how one should think about the role of genes thought of as coding for specific traits in environments where the trait is completely irrelevant. Crow, for example, asks us to consider this puzzle from *Drosophila* bred to be resistant to DDT: "what were the genes that detoxify DDT doing before DDT was introduced?" (1986, 113). Even without being able to provide an adequate general answer, however, we can note that the environmental significance (the real social significance) of homosexuality creates an opportunity for genetic effects where none might have existed before.[16]

We might wonder if, for example, there might actually have been a bio-logically discoverable difference between men in classic Athens who enjoyed being penetrated in anal sex and those who did not. Certainly such "research" would have seemed very natural to the ancient Greeks (see Laqueur 1990, 44 and 258, n. 58). But so far at least, no such differences have been found among the members of the gay subcultures in our culture.[17] Indeed, even trying to find a biological "cause" for, say, heterosexual men who enjoy having their anuses manipulated (digitally or otherwise) during sex would be considered bizarre in the extreme. In this way, I am suggesting, our lack of interest in specific sexual tastes probably results in some of those tastes being somewhat more fluid, or at least far less rigid than they would have been for at least some of the ancient Greeks. This seems especially likely, for example, with respect to the passive/active role in sex and the penetrating/penetrated dichotomy. Our decoupling of hierarchical political position from sexual position permits us to unself-consciously partake in various sexual activities that would have been diametrically opposite to the Greeks. Even so, Hamer notes that the homosexual men in his study "exhibited a more flexible and diverse repertoire of sexual activities and desires" than the heterosexual men in the study (see Hamer and Copeland 1994, 168–69).

Appiah's hope seems to be, similarly, that by decoupling one's sexuality from grand life-scripts, one will be able to live one's life in a less restricted way; one will have more choices available, and more range in which personal tastes may play a role (Appiah 1994, 162–63; see also Faderman 1994). Insofar as this is a legitimate goal, searches for genetic or other biological associations with homosexuality—or for that matter heterosexuality—that are supposed to reveal something about its "causes," or indeed searches for biological correlates to a desire to be penetrated anally, will seem worrisome.[18]

Such searches cannot reveal the causal roles of any genes found without far more research into the developmental pathways they are implicated in, and that research is, at best, difficult to pursue in humans. However, they *can* make the formulation of the trait in question seem more stable, more inevitable, than the history of the trait or the differences in its expression cross-culturally would suggest. And that, in turn, could well make the trait more fixed as a category of thought and behavior, in a way that will seem problematic to those people who think different formulations would be associated with important aspects of human flourishing.

CHAPTER 7
ON THE MEDICALIZATION OF MOOD-AFFECTIVE DISORDERS: ANTIDEPRESSANTS AND THE HERITABILITY OF DEPRESSION AND TEMPERAMENT

Locating Depression

If the hackneyed "nature versus nurture" debate were applied to the causal history of clinical depression, we would on the one hand have an argument that some people are *born* depressed and on the other hand an argument that some people are *made* depressed by the environments they face or grow up in. While no researcher frames issues in this "either-or" way anymore, many would now agree that depression is at least in part the result of poor luck in the genetic lottery; some people, in other words, are born prone to depression, and the environment merely brings that tendency out in those people (see Platt and Bach 1997 for a discussion of nature versus nurture debates, questions, and common mistakes in psychology). Even those researchers who stress the role of "temperament" in depression make the link out to be direct. Some people, on this view, have temperaments that are "more sensitive," either to environmental stresses or more generally, and these people end up depressed in large part *because* their temperaments predispose them to depression.

The standard story that has grown out of the treatment of depression and research into its causes might be summed up as follows: Some people are genetically predisposed toward biochemical brain disorders that result in depression. When these disorders occur, depression results, and the correct cure is to fix the biochemical disorder. Modern antidepressants do that, so the argument goes, and do it without very many nasty side effects. Depression is a disease of the individual's brain chemistry, and is therefore best fixed through individually directed medical (biochemical) intervention.

But how fair is this story to the complexities of the research that has actually been done on the causal history of depression and, more generally, temperament and personality? Here I argue that, at best, it is not very fair; that it hides major aspects of the research, and furthermore, that these aspects are important to the way we view depression in society. One of these points is again a technical point about what studies of heritability actually show. Even if depression is highly heritable in the technical sense, recall that this means *not* that some people are born prone to depression *simpliciter*, but rather that within a certain population within a certain environment, much of the differences in rates of depression may be "attributed" to genetics (in the technical sense described in chapter 3). So even if some people in our current society are born prone to depression, the studies we have now show only that they do so only *within* the environments in which the study was done. Changing the environment may well result in the heritability changing—perhaps dropping to zero, perhaps increasing. Again, without knowing the reaction norms for the traits in question in the environments envisioned, there is no way of saying which (see chapter 3).

More importantly, I'll argue that those researchers who have been concentrating on the links between temperament and depression have focused too exclusively on the most obvious of pathways between the two. The move from the claim that much of the heritability of depression can be explained by the heritability of temperament to the claim that temperaments are therefore to blame for depression is made much too quickly. Looked at another way, this same relationship can make the environment out to play a much more important role in the development of depression. While changing the environment in such a way that fewer people end up depressed may not, in the end, prove feasible or even possible, the causal pathway of the disease would, on this view, end up having to talk about the relationship between people and their environments. Depression would cease to be strictly about individuals with predispositions to poor brain chemistry (either directly or because of their "temperaments"), and would be about the relationships people have to their (social) environments. This is a very different approach, and one that, at least in principle, could be seen as empowering.

The Heritability and Heterogeneity of Affective Disorders

The mood-affective disorders are generally divided into two major categories: depression, including both single major episodes and unipolar depression, and bipolar disorders, where depression alternates with manic elevations of mood. However, these categories fail to capture the complex relationships these disorders have to each other, nor do they do justice to the variety of affective disorders. The relationship between the different affective disorders is still contentious, but a variety of techniques for assessing the degree of relatedness between the different affective disorders are converging on the assertion that there is a relationship between the various forms of mild unipolar depression, cyclic depressions, bipolar affective disorders, and, perhaps, certain classes of obsessive-compulsive disorders and certain forms of schizophrenia. Those techniques seem to imply that mood-affective disorders centered on single major depressive episodes are less related or not related to those others.

The heritability of both unipolar depressive disorders (depression) and bipolar depression (manic depression) has been studied by twin, adoption, and first-degree relative studies. In the case of unipolar depressive disorders, specifically those involving a single major episode, the studies have yielded somewhat confused results, with twin studies yielding higher, and sometimes much higher, apparent heritability estimates than adoption studies, but in any event it is often claimed that these studies do seem to point toward there being some genetic influence (see Plomin et al. 1990, 377–78, 394; Plomin et al. 1997, 178–82). Twin studies of bipolar depression seem to point to a very high heritability; however, as with unipolar depression, adoption studies yield lower estimates for heritability than do twin studies, and so the twin results must be approached with caution (see Plomin et al. 1990, 138–39). And again, recall that heritability estimates in human populations are never particularly reliable, and that heritability is often misinterpreted.

The attempt to find genes linked to affective disorders, though, has proven frustrating. Two early studies purporting to show linkages, one in Israeli families and another in Older Order Amish, were both retracted relatively quickly (see Plomin et al. 1990, 379; Horgan 1993, 125). While no recent studies have claimed to find a gene associated with depression *simpliciter* (see Plomin et al. 1997, 183), there has been a report of the discovery of a gene associated with the level of one's "anxiety" (see Lesch et al. 1996; and Hamer and Copeland 1998) which, it is argued, is a related trait (see below). Further, while some of these same studies have seemed to imply that bipolar depression is distinct from unipolar depression in that a high familial incidence of one does not imply an increased familial incidence of the other, other research has suggested that while unipolar depression with single major episodes may be distinct from bipolar depression, milder forms of unipolar depression, and cyclic unipolar depression may both be related to bipolar depression, and perhaps to schizophrenia, both clinically and genetically (see Kramer 1993, 166ff., 319, 347ff.; and Nigg and Goldsmith 1994, 357ff.; but see Moldin et al. 1991, 223–25).

Part of the problem is that, traditionally, one way of distinguishing and grouping psychological disorders is by what sort of treatment they respond to. However, as different treatments tend to work on/affect different purported classes of psychological disorders, grouping this way yields unstable groups, as drugs affect relatively larger or smaller classes. The relatively recent increase in the use of SSRIs (serotonin selective reuptake inhibitors) has focused attention on the relatively larger groups, as drugs in this class seem useful for everything from mild depressions to obsessive-compulsive behavior disorders (see Kramer 1993).

Affective Disorders and Temperament

In any event, while the claimed relationship among various forms of affective disorders is by no means certain, it at least provides an entry into an even more contentious area of research—that which explores the relationship between temperament, broadly construed, and the affective disorders. Relatively recent research is increasingly seen as pointing toward depression, neuroticism, and anxiety being "linked" (see for example Watson and Clark 1994; Hamer and Copeland 1998; McGuire and Troisi 1998). Watson et al. (1994) suggest that high correlations between various "dysphoric mood states" and "dysfunctional cognitive schema" are the result of their being "a single, more general construct," that being, loosely, a personality or temperament type; in this case, the more general construct in question is a disposition to neuroticism and "negative affect" (Watson et al. 1994, 29).

However, it is this very relationship that is problematic, for, despite the high correlations, the causal pathways are not at all transparent. Carey and DiLalla (1994) attempt a model-fitting analysis on three strong hypotheses: namely that it is the personality types that cause the disorders, it is the disorders that result in the creation of the personality types, and that some underlying phenotypic trait is responsible for both. However, insofar as their attempt at model fitting revealed anything, it was that none of those models were particularly well supported by the data they used (Carey and DiLalla 1994, 41ff.). McGuire and Troisi, however, suggest that their own research implies that the personality or temperament type associated with "social inhibition" predates the emergence of depressive characteristics, and hypothesize that social inhibition is, in fact, a causal factor in depression, at least in the women McGuire and Troisi studied (see Kramer 1993, 167–72, 348–49 for early reports on this research; McGuire and Troisi 1998, 161–67 for its development). Hamer and Copeland (1998) also follow this model, and it is also suggested by the analysis of depression and stressful life events that Kendler (1998) and Kendler and Karkowski-Shuman (1997) put forward.

An added complexity is that the studies of the heritability of temperament, irrespective of affective disorders, have convinced many researchers in human behavior genetics that "temperament" is a highly heritable and stable trait. Kagan's work on early predictors of inhibited and uninhibited personality types in children is often cited as particularly interesting (see Hamer and Copeland 1998, 63–65). Kagan found a significant correlation between physiological traits and inhibition level, especially in the high correlation between highly "inhibited" personality types and the cluster of blue eyes, pale skin, susceptibility to allergies, a tall, thin physique, narrow facial structure, asymmetries in facial temperature, and relatively high heart rates (see Kagan 1994, 170–236).[1] Using the results of several twin studies, Kagan reports broad-sense heritability of personality type (inhibited or uninhibited) of around .5, and the heritability of extreme personality types, those inhibited and uninhibited personality types that were more than one standard distribution from the norm, at between .7 and .9 (1994, 167–68), although he is (rightly) somewhat cautious about interpreting these results (1994, 166–67; note though that Hamer and Copeland [1998] feel comfortable citing his estimate of .7–.9 with few disclaimers). Carey and DiLalla (1994) report that twin studies of the heritability of personality have converged on heritability estimates of .4–.6 (33). However, as with depression, among other traits, adoption studies have yielded more mixed results, pointing toward a lower bound of perhaps .3 and an upper bound of perhaps .6 (Carey and DiLalla 1994, 33–34). As always with heritability estimates in humans, some degree of skepticism is advisable.

Given the correlations between personality type and mood-affective disorders, and the high heritability of both, it is natural to wonder how much of the correlation can be accounted for by the heritability. Carey and DiLalla, citing one of the few estimates made for this, claim that some 60 percent of the correlation of neuroticism and anxiety in the women they consider can be accounted for by the heritability of the two traits. Hamer and Copeland argue that for the extreme end of the "inhibited" spectrum, the covariance of depression and inhibition can be *entirely* accounted for by their sharing the same genetic etiology (1998, 68). It should be noted that the data that Carey and DiLalla use, unlike the data used by Kagan and the data used by Hamer, do not distinguish between the heritability of extreme and more normal personality types, and so it is unclear how to account for the different interpretations of the data.

On Treating Temperament

There is, then, at least some evidence for there being some relationship, perhaps a quite complex one, between personality and the mood-affective disorders. Clark et al. (1994) suggest that the large role personality seems to play in mood-affective disorders has implications for the treatment of the latter. They wonder if it might be possible to directly treat underlying personality traits, such as those highly correlated with depression, with the hope that this will prove more effective than the treatment of the disorders themselves; that is, they hint that treating the temperament or personality associated with depression would be more effective than focusing on the particular depressive episodes or cycles (see Clark et al. 1994, 113–14).

To a certain extent, some researchers believe that this is already happening. Kramer (1993) contends that one of the effects of SSRIs is to create less inhibited personalities, and that at least part of the effectiveness of treatments based on these drugs can be traced to different relationships patients with their newly less inhibited personality types have with the world. Kramer argues that the patients' depression is reduced at least in part by the increased social rewards garnered by their decreased inhibitions, increased willingness to take risks, and the like (see Kramer 1993, esp. 182–84).

Whether or not this is really the way SSRIs achieve even part of their therapeutic results, the implication that it might be is itself intriguing. Further, that Clark et al. consider temperament a proper place for therapeutic intervention can be seen as pointing in a direction for future pharmacological work. But of course, the idea that temperament and other aspects of overall personality structure are the sorts of things that ought to be viewed as amenable to treatment raises further questions.

If the high correlation of inhibited personality types to mood-affective disorders (especially depression) is, even in part, due to the relationship the temperament has with the rewards available in the environment, changing the temperament represents only one of the ways of breaking the low-reward cycle. Because, after all, it is not a given that inhibited temperament types are going to be associated with low social rewards;

indeed, it has been suggested that in other times, and in other cultures, more social rewards may have accrued to more inhibited temperament types (see Kramer 1993, 269ff. and Kagan 1994, 250ff.; Lewis-Fernández and Kleinman 1994 make a related point). While it might seem improbable, perhaps for what might be termed practical reasons, changing the *environment* to one more suited to the temperament would, it could be argued, achieve much the same results as changing the temperament to suit the environment.

Depression as Disease: Treatment, Pharmacology, Genetics, and Temperament

Before attempting to problematize the current stories told about the causes of and proper level at which to view the treatment of depression, I'd like to inject a note of caution. In critiquing these approaches, I hope it is obvious that I do not mean to suggest that depression is not a serious problem for those people suffering from it; nor do I mean to suggest that drug-based therapies are always, or even often, inappropriate. In suggesting here that certain ways of treating depression — in both the literal sense of the medical treatment offered and the metaphoric sense of the discourse we permit to surround depression — are strikingly problematic when viewed through a certain lens, I am for the most part concerned with the theoretical background of the stories told. I am concerned, again, with the way that, for example, successful drug-based treatments interact with the discourse surrounding a depressive episode to hide the importance of the environment, at least in many cases. This should *not* be interpreted as an attack on current *treatments*, but rather, if anything, as a call for a more cautious language pending further research.

In any event, most diagnosed mood-affective disorders are currently treated with a combination of traditional psychiatric therapy and antidepressant drugs, although the popularity of drug-based therapies without traditional psychotherapy is perhaps increasing. Once depression is made out to be a disease, a biochemical dysfunction of some sort, the natural place to intervene is taken to be at the biochemical level.[2] In a sense, the articulation of mental illness as disease, albeit a disease of subtle brain chemistries, carries with itself it the medicalization of depression, for it is technoscientific medicine that is responsible for the treatment of diseases, and which has, traditionally, done so invasively.

In this case, doing so has created an atmosphere in which mood-affective disorders are made out to be, for the most part, the problem of the patient. The trend toward seeing mood-affective disorders as part of an array of heritable characteristics has encouraged this view. While "environmental stressors" are habitually mentioned, mood-affective disorders are increasingly seen as the result of a genetic predisposition to biochemical disorders of the brain. Insofar as the environment is held to have a role in influencing mood-affective disorders, it is generally considered to be that which brings the predisposition to the fore, that which merely permits a problem that was, in effect, already there to be displayed.

Given this view, a tendency to favor drug-based treatments is understandable. If the problem is a problem of brain chemistry, and it is possible to modify brain chemistry directly, doing so is a natural move. The assumption that brain chemistry is the proper place for intervention to take place is reinforced by fact that, very often at least, modifying brain chemistry does have a positive effect on the condition to be treated, albeit usually one with a string of not insignificant side effects. Indeed, when drug-based therapies fail to work, this can be blamed not on their failure to cure the illness (depression) but rather the patient's inability to deal with his or her new condition of health; in this view, traditional psychotherapeutic methods can be a useful tool for helping patients deal with their new "healthy" state, although not for curing a disease (see for example Kramer 1993, 291–93).

Part of the effect of this transformation has been the creation of a situation in which a patient's ability to make certain claims about her condition is diminished. If one is told that one's depression is the result of a genetic predisposition to an biochemical problem, one's ability to claim that it is one's environment that is problematic is cut off. The success of drug-based treatments may further limit the patient's potential to critique her environment as at fault.[3]

Neither the heritability of mood-affective disorders nor the success of drug-based treatments in affecting the course of mood-affective disorders should, however, be taken to imply that the environment is not playing a vital role. Heritability, again, is a measure that only makes sense given a particular population within a particular range of environments. How particular genotypes will interact with particular environments to produce phenotype is, again, not currently predictable without doing the sorts of experiments that give rise to norm of reaction tables—again, these are impossible in humans (see chapter 3). The success in modifying brain chemistry via pharmaceuticals does not imply that other approaches to changing the relationship that the patient has with the world, such as changing the environment, would not have been successful.

Consider again the hypothesis that at least some of the heritability of depression is the result of the heritability of temperaments that make the sort of behavior rewarded in this culture less easily engaged in. Imagine further that at least a portion of the success of certain classes of antidepressants in treating these cases results from their changing the temperaments of the individuals in question to ones that result in more highly rewarded behavior patterns; that is, they modify personalities so that engaging in more highly rewarded behavior patterns is easier or more comfortable for the people involved. In this case, I take it, the claim that these people are suffering from a mood-affective disorder because they are genetically predisposed to a certain class of biochemical brain disorders is true only in the most perverse sense. It is at least just as accurate to describe their condition as their finding themselves in a culture that does not reward the majority of the behavior patterns they find comfortable and natural, and that this has resulted in their having to act in ways they find intensely unpleasant and stressful, as well as their not getting their share of social rewards. On this description, it can be thought that the society, by not providing the cultural space necessary for a significant portion of its members to flourish, is at least as much at fault as the depressed individuals' genes and brain chemistries.

Even under this description, the suggested treatment for depression might remain the same—pharmacological, perhaps combined with traditional psychiatric therapy. This is because it is obviously very difficult to make significant changes in our social environments in directed ways, and further, we as yet have no idea just what kinds of changes would be effective! But there is a clear and important distinction to be made here nonetheless. Under one description, the patient is told that her depression is the result of a heritable biochemical disorder, and therefore she should take some antidepressant to "fix" the problem with her brain chemistry, and thereby circumvent the disorder. Under the other description, the patient is told that his depression is the result of his having had the misfortune of being born into a culture that doesn't respect or reward the temperamental qualities that, in this culture, he had a genetic predisposition toward and did in fact develop, and that he should therefore take an antidepressant in the hope of its changing his temperament to one that will permit him to garner more social rewards with less unpleasantness. The latter description at least raises the issue of the quality of the environments, both social and otherwise, that we find ourselves in, and directly confronts the attempt at fitting individuals into a society and culture with which they might not be at all comfortable.

A common reaction to these sorts of suggestions is to claim that there are people for whom drug-based therapies represent the only hope of alleviating their depression, and that there are clearly some people for whom any change in their environment would be ineffective. I take it that this is a different claim from the claim that there are genetic dispositions that, in any environment, would yield depression. The latter claim is not at all supported by, for example, studies of identical twins, where the correlations are always less than one; that is, there are no mood-affective disorders such that if one identical twin gets it, the other is certain to. However, I take the claim under discussion to be that for at least some cases of depression, once the genetic, in combination with some environmental influences, has led to the biochemical disorder, only interventionist biochemical fixes can repair it. I find this claim both shocking and deeply disturbing, as I cannot believe that the people who make this claim are thinking of any research that has been done on the topic, for the simple reason that there has been none or next to none. I have never seen nor heard of any research on attempts to use radical environmental change to alleviate depression, and am forced to take the ubiquity of the claim that any such attempts would surely fail to be evidence that, within our society, the biochemical line on depression is already firmly entrenched. The closest suggestion I have been able to find is the obvious fact that without treatment, individuals suffering from severe mood-affective disorders who are institutionalized don't get better simply because of their institutionalization, but I do not think of this as the sort of environmental change we would expect to have a positive influence on mood-affective disorders—indeed, rather the opposite.[4] Far from there being persuasive research on the topic, I can think of no hard evidence one could even provide for the view that some significant portion of people suffering from mood-affective disorders would not be benefited by some radical change in their environment. A related problem can be seen by asking, How many environments would one have to try before being able to legitimately claim that no *conceivable* environment would be effective?[5]

More importantly, perhaps, such an objection misses the point completely. Again, recall that many biologists now believe that most phenotypes are the result of complex interactions, including those between the genes (epistasis) and those between genes and the environment. Many of these complex interactions occur during the ill-understood developmental process. It may now be impossible to alleviate the sort of mood-affective disorders that come from our society's lack of cultural space for certain temperaments without the use of drugs to directly modify brain chemistry; this does not imply, however, that had such cultural space existed, there would have been any depression to treat at all. Failing to provide the cultural or social room for the temperaments that some significant portion of the population finds itself with might well be regarded as a biting criticism of a society even if, or perhaps especially if, those people who already find themselves suffering because of this are now unable to be helped without direct chemical intervention.

In the end it may well prove to be impossible to create social systems that provide the sort of cultural space necessary for *every* temperament type to flourish. However, the suggestion that it is still very different to point toward the interaction of a social system and a temperament as a location for causal responsibility than it is to point toward a genetic disorder *simpliciter*, is still, I think, telling. In the discourse that surrounds contemporary research, one can clearly see the assumption that the environment is at best secondary, that trying to change it is useless, and that drug-based treatments are the obvious solution to psychological problems. This clearly points toward a system unwilling to even consider the modifications that might permit more rather than fewer temperament types to flourish, whether or not such modifications should prove possible.

Biochemistry, Genetics, and the Environment

The above section attempted to problematize one of the popular current ways of conceptualizing and treating mood-affective disorders. However, the narrow focus on claimed genetic etiologies for depression, or temperaments associated with depression, shifted somewhat to a more general account of the *location* of the causal basis of depression. Here, I attempt to pull these threads together and display their relationship more perspicuously.

First, note that an emphasis on the biochemical and an emphasis on the genetic share the property that they make the condition out to be *internal* to the patient, both in terms of cause and in terms of what the condition actually consists in. Making a condition and a treatment out to be internal to the patient is an inherently stabilizing move.[6] Once a genetic explanation is offered, and any plausible sounding pathway proposed, the opportunities for claiming that there are other ways of approaching the problem are radically curtailed. A mood-affective disorder ceases to be about a set of difficulties between a person and his environment, and becomes a disease, a problem with the internal functioning of that person.

Indeed, even those views of depression that link it to temperament usually make the depression out to follow directly from the temperament, which is considered to be the thing "under genetic control" (see Kendler 1998; Hamer and Copeland 1998; McGuire and Troisi 1998). If the environment comes into the story at all, it can also be made out to be under a form of "indirect" genetic control; people with certain temperaments are more likely to "select" themselves into certain environments than people with different temperaments (see Kendler 1998; Kendler and Karkowski-Shuman 1997). But generally the link between the temperament and depression is thought to be fairly direct—certain temperaments are supposed to be more "sensitive" and therefore susceptible to depression. Various kinds of evolutionary storytelling, usually involving kinds of "pleiotropy" and other genetic constraints, are put into play to explain why so many people are born predisposed to temperaments that cause them "to feel anxious, depressed, and pessimistic" (as Hamer and Copeland would have it: 1998, 81). The general claim is that the same "genes" that result in an anxious temperament do other things as well, things that have a positive evolutionary value; so for example Hamer suggests that the genes responsible for anxious temperaments may also increase sex drive (see Hamer and Copeland 1998, 81–82; McGuire and Troisi 1998, 161–63). Again, the final "location" of the cause of the disease in this story is a genetic predisposition that would, it is to be supposed, show in at least many environments.

As drug-based treatments become ever more sophisticated, the claim that their success shows that it was the brain chemistry all along that was at fault becomes ever more believable. With this conviction that biochemistry is both the culprit and the place at which to generate cures comes a decreasing sophistication in dealing with other potential sources of the alleviation of the psychological pain associated with mood-affective disorders, as drugs become the first-line treatment and, at least partially because they are the first thing tried, the treatment with the highest success rate. The story that is told surrounding depression, then, becomes one of genes, brain chemistry, and the clever pharmacologists whose drugs can alleviate those biochemical problems the unfortunate person's genotype has left him with.

The emphasis on the genes as the ultimate source for behavior hides those environmental factors that are significant. Even where a genetic influence exists, the pathway by which it works remains, for the most part, unexplored. As above, different pathways can have very different implications for the sort of story that is to be told around an illness—it can be the difference between making an affective disorder out to be primarily a mismatch of social order and temperament, or to be a matter of raw biochemical disease.

Again, a slightly different story involving a mismatch between temperaments and social environments would have very different implications for explaining, if not necessarily for treating, depression. Indeed, such a story would permit the easy explanation of the rise in rates of depression in developed nations, something a straightforwardly genetic etiology has some trouble explaining (noted by Plomin et al. 1997, 178, and Hamer and Copeland 1998, 85). Of course there isn't really any very good evidence one way or the other now—both the "direct" model and the "socially mediated" model of the relationship of temperament to depression can account for much of the data available (much of which is pretty questionable anyway—see Platt and Bach 1997; Bailey 1997; and chapter 3). But the two stories have very different implication for understanding mood-affective disorders, and different implications for thinking about the society we live in and its relationship to mood-affective disorders.

With the current emphasis on the heritable, on the genetic simply construed, rides the unquestioned assumption that the environment we find ourselves in, and in which we generate heritability estimates, is the only one available to us, the only one it makes sense to think about. As heritability tells us nothing about what the results of changing the environment might be, to study heritability at all, to take heritability estimates at all seriously, is to assume an environment that we are unable or unwilling to change (for more on this topic, see chapter 10). While the claim that psychology, and medicine in general, are forces of stability in society— that, in other words, they are technologies of the status quo—has been much scoffed at of late, the excitement with which the medical and psychiatric professions have embraced heritability studies should perhaps give us pause (see Platt and Bach 1997, 138ff. for a critique of heritability studies in psychology).

Once the story of mood-affective disorders as a class of biochemically based diseases resulting from genetic conditions becomes entrenched, and once the pharmaceutical treatments of these so-called diseases become sophisticated and popular enough, no other stories can be told. The conviction of so many people that antidepressants are, for at least some people afflicted with mood-affective disorders, not merely the only practical, but the only possible source of help dramatically displays this trend. The genetic becomes not necessarily the unchangeable, but that which we must change in a bold interventionist way (see chapter 2). The environment becomes the passive participant in the process of disease formation; and changing the environment ends up being an option that is not even discussable, let alone discussed.

CHAPTER 8
BORN TO BE FAT? CULTURE AND THE MEANING OF WEIGHT

Health and the Ideal Weight

Obtaining the "ideal" body type is an obsession in contemporary American culture; this obsession is most pronounced, and has the most widespread destructive results, in American women. The ideal body type in American culture is, it need hardly be mentioned, "extremely thin [and] physically fit" (Brownell 1991, 1), although, again, standards for men have been somewhat more tolerant of body types other than the radically thin than they have been for women. All this is well-known, but it is worth noting just how radical the obsession with weight loss is. Brownell notes, in "Dieting and the Search for the Perfect Body: Where Physiology and Culture Collide," that as of the late 1980s, Americans were spending well over thirty billion dollars a year on weight loss–related products, specifically "diet foods, programs, books, etc." (1991, 1; see also Barinaga 1995, 475). By 1998 the figure had climbed to around fifty billion dollars a year (Kassirer and Angell 1998, 52). While this obsession with weight loss fits in well with some comments by the medical profession about, for example, obesity being the "second leading cause of preventable death in America" (Koop, quoted by Kassirer and Angell 1998, 52; see also below), the money spent "treating" obesity is rarely connected to clear health benefits, and in any event is mostly wasted from any standpoint (Kassirer and Angell 1998, 52).

But the pursuit of this "ideal" body type is not only, or even primarily, about health. Rather, it is wrapped up in a complex set of symbolic relationships involving cultural beliefs about the value of "self-control, hard work, and the delay of gratification" and the relationship these are thought to have to being thin and fit (Brownell 1991, 4). Given this, people considered overweight by contemporary standards find themselves enmeshed in a set of beliefs involving their being "indulgent, lazy, and lacking control" (Brownell 1991, 4; see also Kassirer and Angell 1998, 52–53).

Behind such relationships, however, lurk assumptions about the plasticity of individual body types (Brownell 1991, 2). In order for such links between weight and notions of self-control and hard work to be coherent, weight must actually be controllable; that is, weight should, for the symbolic relationship to hold, actually be *relatable* to those traits, even if not actually related.

Current medical wisdom, for the most part, holds otherwise. The high heritability of weight, and especially of obesity, the wide range of resting metabolic rates and their relationship to weight, and set point theory have all been used to cast doubt on the notion that obesity is even primarily under the individual's local behavioral control (see Brownell and Wadden 1991, 156; Hamer and Copeland 1998, 245; and below for more details). More to the point, the consistent failure of people to radically alter their weight is ample evidence that doing so is at least extraordinary difficult (see Kassirer and Angell 1998, 52–53). Increasingly, this view has become publicly accepted, at least at the level of conscious discourse, and individuals considered overweight by contemporary standards are not, in general, held to be morally culpable for their condition. Of course, while most people now would not *say* of people they considered overweight that they are lazy, irresponsible, or lack self-control simply as evidenced by their "weight problem," it seems that at least many people would be more inclined to make such judgments of people considered overweight *because*, in a strictly causal sense, the people are overweight. That is, it may be the case that while people are now less inclined to *say* things such as "that person is overweight, so that person must be lazy and irresponsible" when confronted with an overweight person, people are still inclined to *judge* that they are in fact lazy and irresponsible. Certainly, some research points toward judgments of that form being very common in American culture (see for example Patzer 1985 and citations therein).

This change in discourse, however deep it goes, has not done anything to change contemporary standards. While being overweight by contemporary standards is no longer held to be entirely the fault of the individual in any strong moral sense, it is still considered to be a problem, and primarily a problem of the individual. Moreover, obesity has become increasingly sharply defined as a medical problem, and treated as such by the medical profession and the public at large. While it is recognized that people who are overweight are not, in some sense, at fault for their condition, they are still supposed to have a problem, and often a problem in need of medical treatment.

In what follows, I will attempt to bring out just how narrow this view of "obesity" is. The medical community has created "obesity" as a condition, and, implicitly, the "obese" person as a type of patient. It has done this despite the widespread acknowledgment that obesity isn't really *a* condition at all, but a heterogeneous class of conditions, some of which involve no increased medical, or, more broadly, health risks whatsoever. Indeed, the only thing that links these very different conditions is the social construction of the sufferers as "overweight" by contemporary standards, standards that other cultures regard as absurd, and indeed that have no long history in our own culture.

The primary point of this section will be to explore the way in which the medicalization of a condition, while often looking like a progressive step, can have the unintended consequence of fixing that condition as problematic. Once obesity becomes a genetic and metabolic liability, rather than a personal failing, the search for medical "treatments" automatically follows. While no "magic bullet" has been discovered yet, the hope for a simple drug-based therapy for obesity continues, and "breakthroughs" are announced regularly, though so far none has panned out (see below; and Barinaga 1995; Pelleymounter et al. 1995; Halaas et al. 1995; Campfield et al. 1995; Barinaga 1996). In this way, the medicalization of weight fixes "obesity" as an undesirable condition. Once obesity becomes identified as a treatable medical condition it becomes much more difficult to claim that current standards of weight in, say, American culture are unrealistic, and that a substantial portion of what is currently regarded as "overweight" should be accepted as part of the normal variation in human weights. The medicalization of weight threatens to severely limit the possible discourse surrounding weight; specifically, such a move threatens to exclude the possibility that current medicalized standards of "ideal" weights treat too many perfectly normal, and potentially desirable, body types as being conditions in need of treatment.[1]

In making these points, I do not want to seem to be denying that at least some forms of obesity are associated with serious medical problems, nor do I want to suggest that these forms should remain untreated. Rather, I would like to suggest that the attention in "treating" obesity should be focused almost entirely on the medical well-being, the health and physical comfort of the individuals involved, and that social aspects of weight control should be actively resisted. In part this is because only after the social aspects of weight become a less than determining factor in what counts as "overweight" will an assessment of the real long-term costs and benefits of weight loss be possible, and a social reconceptualization of what it means to be a "normal" weight able to occur.

Defining Obesity

Obesity has been defined in several different ways. The most common but least satisfactory way makes "being obese" out to be having a weight of above a certain percentage of the "desirable body weight" (DBW). The "desirable body weight table" was developed by Metropolitan Life Insurance Company in 1959, based on their actuarial work relating body weight to likely life spans, and, in a slightly modified form, is still in wide use (see Simopoulos 1988; Bray 1987). These tables give the "desirable" range of weights for various heights for men and women. Using a system like this, obesity is naturally defined as being a certain amount "overweight," that is, above the maximum "desirable" weight range. Brownell and Wadden (following other practitioners) suggest the following breakdown into "levels" of obesity: "Level I = 5–20% overweight; Level II = 21 –40%; Level III = 41–100%; Level IV = 100%+" (1991, 161).

Another popular method is to derive a person's "body mass index" (BMI), which is the result of their weight in kilograms divided by the square of their height in meters. The "desirable" BMI is said to be around 21.5 kg/m^2, with a range of 20-25 kg/m^2 considered more or less acceptable. A BMI in excess of 25 is usually thought to represent obesity, and a BMI in excess of 30 extreme obesity (see for example Simopoulos 1988; Jarrett 1988). The BMI is thought to have significance primarily because of its supposed high correlation (.6–.8) with body fat percentage (see Simopoulos 1988, 2–3; Jarrett 1988, Bouchard and Pérusse 1993), which, it is often thought, is the real issue (Simopoulos 1988; Jarrett 1988; Bouchard and Pérusse 1993). When dealing with individuals, it is possible to estimate body fat percentages directly by such techniques as multiple skin-fold thickness tests, weight when immersed in water, the electrical resistance of body parts, and the like (see Jarrett 1988). However, for population samples, especially as used in epidemiological research, such techniques are impossibly unwieldy, forcing the use of such stand-ins as BMIs (Jarrett 1988). But since the correlation between BMI and body fat percentage is known to vary between ethnicities, and may vary based on other factors, extreme caution should be, but often is not, taken when using BMI in epidemiological studies in heterogeneous populations or in making comparisons between populations (see for example Duncan et al. 1995; Wang et al. 1994; Ortiz et al. 1992; and Le Marchand 1991).

Definitions of obesity based directly on body fat percentages usually define obesity as the state of having a body fat content greater than 25 percent of total body weight in males or greater than 30 percent in females (Gray and Bray 1988, 47). The "normal" body fat percentages for young adult males is thought to be around 15–18 percent, and that for young adult females around 20–26 percent (Gray and Bray 1988). Elite athletes often have much lower percentages, with, for example, elite long-distance women runners often having body fat percentages in the range of 10–15 percent (Brownell 1991, 3).

None of these definitions, however, does justice to the heterogeneity of obesity. That a person has been defined as "obese" using any of these definitions gives little clue about his medical condition. Depending on where, for example, the "extra" body fat is carried, the same "level" of obesity can have serious metabolic and medical complications, or, as far as can be determined, none at all (see Després et al. 1992). That is, some people diagnosed as obese have "a cosmetic problem but perhaps not a condition requiring medical intervention" (Després et al. 1992, 165–66). Bouchard and Pérusse present a breakdown of obesity into four types, depending on where the "extra" fat is carried (Bouchard and Pérusse 1993).[2] Such heterogeneity may explain such otherwise baffling results as the lower than average life expectancy of moderately obese people as given by, for example, the Metropolitan Life actuarial tables, and the (preliminary) results that a higher than average number of the longest-lived people are moderately obese and that moderate obesity seems to be correlated with the lowest health risks in the very old (Stini 1991 and Schneider 1994).[3]

Bouchard and Pérusse note that due to the heterogeneity of obesity, "strictly speaking, one should . . . talk about obesities rather than obesity" (Bouchard and Pérusse 1993, 26–27); however, this formulation merely raises the question of why a trait with no medical complications whatsoever should be called "obesity" at all. "Obesity," after all, is a loaded term; it carries meaning, and as a negative label in general use will continue to have negative connotations even if it were to be called, in those cases where it carried no health risks, say, "medically irrelevant obesity." And further, note that it is unclear why we need to pay attention to medically irrelevant weight ranges at all. Why, in other words, does the medical community need a name for a class of weights that have nothing of medical interest in common with one another? Tellingly, in Craddock's discussion of the role of the general practitioner in treating obesity, he notes that some patients seeking advice will have "no obvious medical reasons for losing weight" and yet given the social significance of being "overweight," "it is hard not to accept for treatment a patient who is concerned" about their current weight (1988, 194).

Most discussions of obesity systematically exclude those forms of obesity directly traceable to straightforward metabolic errors (see Gray and Bray 1988, 52–53 for a list of some of these conditions). It should be mentioned, though, *that* such forms are excluded, since, culturally, "obese" carries with it connotations of the sort of extraordinary obesity—"morbid obesity," in the literature—that is often associated with such syndromes. In these syndromes, other medical problems are often extreme. Calling these problems "obesity" is, again, deeply problematic, since their etiologies are so distinct from the "ordinary" forms of obesities usually discussed.

In a sense, this hints at what the best definitions of obesity might entail: an attention to the medical conditions demanding treatment. The heterogeneity of obesity might best be brought out by a consideration of what medical problems a given form of obesity is actually associated with. Those examples of obesity associated with identifiable medical problems, such as hypertension, angina, congestive heart failure, diabetes, osteoarthritis, esophageal reflux, somnolence, cerebrovascular disease, and the like, should certainly be treated (see for example Bray 1987; Jarrett 1988; Gray and Bray 1988; Craddock 1988 for lists of conditions associated with kinds of obesity). But "treating" something as a medical condition—and indeed, starting medical treatments of it—before it is associated with any medical problems should strike us as problematic, especially if it is unclear if the condition will *ever* be associated with any medical problems. Where the "excess" weight doesn't strike the *patient* as a problem, the claim that it is still a disease in need of treatment is especially troublesome (see Brownell and Wadden 1991, 160; see also Helb and Heatherton 1998). (More on this below.)

Genetics and the Etiology of Obesity

Researchers have generated estimates of the heritability of such things as obesity, weight, and body fat, using studies of siblings, twins, and twins reared apart, as well as adoption studies. As is often the case, there is a huge variation in results, with estimates of broad-sense heritability ranging from near zero to almost .9, depending in part on the way the study was framed (Bouchard and Pérusse 1993, 30). Those studies that concentrated on weight *simpliciter* seem to generate numbers ranging from about .4 to about .6 (Plomin et al. 1990, 320–22; Brownell and Wadden 1991;

Bouchard and Pérusse 1993; Allison et al. 1996, and 1994 cite larger numbers for their twin studies, in the .6–.7 range, which Hamer and Copeland 1998 follow). Those studies concentrating on the heritability of body fat percentage seem to generate somewhat lower numbers, in the .2–.3 zone (Bouchard and Pérusse 1993; Després et al. 1992). Those that concentrate on obesity, defined more broadly, have generated numbers closer to .6 (Brownell and Wadden 1991); however, Bouchard and Pérusse argue that once the data are adjusted to reflect age and gender, they do not support any heritability estimates of obesity or weight *simpliciter* in excess of .4 (Bouchard and Pérusse 1993, 31). Bouchard and Pérusse, and Després et al., report that heritabilities for where the "extra" fat is carried (for obesity type, in Bouchard and Pérusse's formulation—see note 2) vary depending on the type of fat. The heritability of subcutaneous fat was estimated as quite low in earlier research (in the .05 range), but more recent work by Pérusse has increased the estimate to perhaps .4 or so for certain sorts of subcutaneous fat (Pérusse et al. 1996). The heritabilities of "deep fat or visceral adipose tissue" (corresponding to type II obesity— see note 2) were estimated as moderately high, perhaps somewhat above .25 (Després et al. 1992, 160–62; Bouchard and Pérusse 1993, 29–32). The large variation in heritability estimates isn't perhaps surprising given the difficulties involved in generating accurate heritability estimates in human populations, and given that heritability estimates are so context dependent in any event (see chapter 3).

What accounts for the heritability of obesity is still an open question.[4] Indeed, given the heterogeneity of the condition, it is unlikely that any single causal explanation will be able to account for all or even most forms of obesity observed. Several different kinds of explanations have been offered, and several different hypothetical mechanisms put forward for investigation. No consensus has yet formed around which are to be preferred.

While little research has been done on the heritability of resting metabolic rates, it is at least a plausible source for some of the heritability of weight in general (see Brownell and Wadden 1991, 155). Again, while little research has been done on the subject, it seems possible that the number of fat cells an individual has, or perhaps an individual's tendency to acquire more, is heritable; as some forms of obesity, especially those associated with early onset, involve individuals having radically elevated numbers of fat cells, this could explain part of the heritability of obesity (Brownell and Wadden 1991, 155–56). A reported but as yet unreplicated molecular finding related to elevated numbers of fat cells has made this mechanism seem more plausible in the case of at least one relatively rare form of massive obesity (see Ristow et al. 1998). Other molecular genetics studies of obesity have met with very limited success; a few linkages have been reported but not replicated in relatively isolated populations, but the genes involved, if they exist at all, have not yet been found nor sequenced (see Bouchard 1997 for a survey).

Set point theory explains the heritability of weight in much broader terms. Primarily, set point theory argues, from the relative stability of weight over time in individuals (Keesey 1978, 524–25) and the smaller than expected gains or losses associated with increases or decreases in caloric intake (Keesey 1988, 88), that body weight in humans is "regulated at a relatively constant level" and that this weight will be "defended against pressure to change" (Brownell and Wadden 1991, 156; see also Keesey 1978, 1988; Kassirer and Angell 1998). As yet, set point theory is still contentious, and even if the theory should turn out to be illuminating, it is unclear if individuals should be thought of as having a set point for their weight, or a set range of weights (see Brownell and Wadden 1991, 156). It is especially unclear that set points are heritable, or even that they are under any nontrivial form of genetic influence; however, should it turn out that human weight is regulated in this fashion, and that set points are heritable, of course at least some forms of obesity would turn out to be heritable in this fashion (Keesey 1978, 526; Keesey 1988, 100). Keesey, though, explicitly notes that only some forms of obesity will be amenable to analysis in terms of a "naturally" elevated set point; other forms of obesity will involve such things as errors in weight regulation such as displaced set points or massively impaired weight-regulatory systems, or massive and long-term environmental disruption, or dietary obesity (Keesey 1988, 100).

Research points toward the conclusion that in the majority of cases of obesity, increased caloric intake is not a factor; indeed, many obese individuals can maintain their weight on *fewer* calories per day than individuals of average weight (Brownell and Wadden 1991, 157). Nor, again in the majority of cases, does the eating "style"—things like the frequency or speed—of obese people differ from that of the average (Brownell and Wadden 1991, 157). Brownell and Wadden note that while *some* obese individuals do overeat, and some have radically different eating habits, including such eating disorders as binge eating, these are, in general, different conditions that must be dealt with on their own terms, and that most cases of obesity will not be amenable to treatment along the lines suggested by these conditions (Brownell and Wadden 1991, 157–58). Except for relatively uncommon sorts of cases where obesity is part of a pattern of psychological problems, obese individuals do not "display any special psychopathology" (Brownell and Wadden 1991, 157). While obese individuals engage in a less than average amount of physical exercise, it is unclear whether this is primarily a cause or an effect of obesity (Brownell and Wadden 1991, 157).

At a broader environmental level, it is often thought that, excepting cases of clear metabolic disorders, there are *dispositions* to become obese that are only expressed under appropriate conditions, conditions that are much more common in affluent modern societies than in, for example, traditional hunter-gatherer societies (Simopoulos 1996, 127–28; Brown and Konner 1987, 32–33; Powers 1988, 35; Bouchard and Pérusse 1993, 28–29, 32). Specifically, the environmental variables at issue are thought to be the switch to relatively high-fat, high-sugar, low-fiber diets and the decrease in physical activity (Brown and Konner 1987, 32–33; Powers 1988, 35; Brownell and Wadden 1991, 154; Nesse and Williams 1995, 147–50). Under conditions of relative abundance and low average rates of physical activity, it is hypothesized, genes that make an individual *susceptible* to obesity will be expressed relatively more often (Simopoulos 1996, 128; Bouchard and Pérusse 1993, 28–29; Hamer and Copeland 1998, 247 –48). Evolutionary explanations are proffered to explain why the tendencies exist at all; generally, the argument is that in pre-agricultural populations, the ability to put on weight during times of relative plenty would have been advantageous, but that this tendency is problematic in a culture where for most people continually acquiring sufficient calories is not generally difficult (see for example Hamer and Copeland 1998, 243; Nesse and Williams 1995, 147–50).

The Social Construction of Ideal Weight

America's obsession with, at least for women, very low body weights (best summed up in the only slightly ironic saying "you can never be too thin or too rich") is a relatively recent phenomenon. Throughout much of the history of Western Europe, it is thought, the standards for female beauty pushed up against what would now be regarded as rather serious obesity (BMIs of around 30) (Brownell 1991, 2–3; Powers 1988, 27–30; Beumont 1988, 44). And in the United States, the ideal weight for females has fluctuated quite a bit over quite short time periods. Powers (1988) points out that Marilyn Monroe would today be considered on rather the high side of normal weight and body fat percentage (with a BMI above that given by the Metropolitan Insurance ideals), and certainly not as having anything like an ideal body type in terms of body fat percentage (see also Brownell 1991). It is now widely recognized that current American cultural ideals for women are actually well below those weights associated with the fewest health problems and lowest mortality rates (Powers 1988, 29–30); indeed, the original Metropolitan Insurance Ideal Weights have been revised upward, in reflecting increased health risks associated with the lower ends of the original ideal weight ranges (Powers 1988 29-30). On the other hand, some recent research has been interpreted by some people as implying that *very* low BMIs are associated with the lowest morbidity risk in women once those with fluctuating weights are excluded (see Manson 1995). In any event, Brownell notes that current standards for "the aesthetic ideal" in women require body fat percentages of less than half what is generally considered a normal level (Brownell 1991, 4). Cross-cultural studies show wide variation in preferred body types, with what American culture would consider "moderately fat" being the ideal at least relatively often (Brown and Konner 1987, 41–42; Klein 1996; see also Stevens et al. 1994 on the heterogeneity of views of weight and attractiveness among elderly women from different ethnic backgrounds in the United States).

Given the relative stability of long-term body weight in at least the environments of contemporary culture, most people's efforts to achieve the current ideal weight in American culture end in failure (Kassirer and Angell 1998, 52; Barinaga 1995, 475; Brownell 1991, 8; Brownell and Wadden 1991, 160–61). Attempts, combined with these failures, result in "weight cycling," a greater than average fluctuation of body weight now widely recognized as unhealthy (see Brownell 1991, 9; Brownell and Wadden 1991, 157–58; see Itoh et al. 1996 for various definitions of weight cycling). Wide variations in an individual's weight have been correlated with coronary heart disease and increased risk for mortality in general (see Itoh et al. 1996, 1996; Jeffery 1996; see Muls et al. 1995; Brownell 1991, 9; and Brownell and Wadden 1991, 157–58 for summaries of past studies). While Brownell notes that it is "not possible to point to specific negative effects [of dieting] at this time . . . much of the existing literature suggests there may be negative effects, including increased risk for morbidity and mortality" and that there is, therefore, "reason for concern regarding the high rates of dieting produced by cultural pressures to be thin" (Brownell 1991, 9; see also Powers 1988, esp. 35–37).

Indeed, it is unclear how much of the excess morbidity and mortality associated with obesity can be explained by the increased morbidity and mortality associated with weight cycling and dieting. Very little work has been done on this topic, but it is likely that extreme weight cycling and dieting are highly correlated with being overweight by contemporary standards. Even if it should turn out that people diagnosable as obese diet no more frequently than the rest of the population, something that seems prima facie unlikely, their weight assuredly varies more, at least in absolute terms, than those of their thinner counterparts. Note too that in the Nurses' Health Study, where the data are often interpreted to show that, barring illness or smoking, thinner simply is healthier, those women who did not have weights that had been relatively stable were excluded (see Manson et al. 1995). It would be illuminating to compare the morbidity and mortality rates of the women in that study whose weights were unstable against those that were stable for a given average BMI. Until some headway has been made in resolving these issues, it is reasonable to doubt both the most radical claims made about the health advantages of extremely low BMIs and the most radical claims made about the extreme health disadvantages of mild obesity (such as, for example, those that appear in Jarrett 1988; Bray 1987; Simopoulos 1987, 1988; Gray and Bray 1988; Barinaga 1995; Manson et al. 1995; and Jung 1997; see also Kassirer and Angell 1998; Brownell 1991; and Brownell and Wadden 1991). It is suggestive that even in clinical contexts where specific instances of obesity have been associated with a specific health problem, relatively small weight losses often have profound health benefits. These small weight losses not only leave patients above the current cultural ideal, but often still solidly diagnosable as "obese"; however, the health benefits of these small losses are often as profound as those associated with larger weight losses, and these small losses are much more likely to be maintained (see Kassirer and Angell 1998; see also Brownell and Wadden 1991, 151ff. for a review of some of the literature on this topic).

Jarrett, in his "Epidemiological Studies in Obesity" notes that conclusions about the relationship of mortality and morbidity to obesity drawn from studies done in one population cannot be generalized to other populations (1988, 17). The simplest reason for this is that given the heterogeneity of obesity, it is unclear from the results of a single population study whether the results will hold for other populations. Since the relationship between obesity in the population studied and other environmental variables cannot be well determined, making accurate predictions about other populations will be difficult if not impossible. Smoking, for example, has an important but complicated effect on obesity, especially on the relationship between obesity and various forms of coronary heart disease; these complicated effects are still being explored (Jarrett 1988, 17, 19; Simopoulos 1988, 9; Gray and Bray 1988, 54). Cross-cultural studies paint a confusing picture of the relationship between obesity and all-cause mortality and morbidity (see Jarrett 1988, 17ff. for a literature review). Some cross-cultural studies show a clear relationship, generally a J-shaped curve, with mortality and morbidity increasing at both extremes of the BMI spectrum; other studies show no general relationship at all between BMI and mortality and morbidity, once age and gender have been taken into account (see Jarrett 1988, 19; also Schneider 1994).

If we take obesity to be a medical condition involving, at the very least, increased health risks, then what society a given particular weight or BMI occurs in may strongly affect whether that weight/BMI should be regarded as "obese." That is, in some environments a BMI that in contemporary American society is associated with increased health risk may not represent a medical condition at all. In cultures where there is no clear relationship between what in the United States is called obesity and medical problems, calling people with these increased body fat percentages "obese" should strike us as problematic. This is especially striking if, in the given culture, what contemporary American culture would call moderate obesity is a preferred body type (BMIs in the 25–35 range are common in many countries). To treat people from such cultures, or indeed many of the people still in such cultures, as if they had a clear medical problem in need of treatment would, I think, be at best misguided.

Brownell and Wadden, in their "Heterogeneity of Obesity: Fitting Treatments to Individuals," introduce the concept of "reasonable weight" as opposed to "ideal weight" as a way of dealing with some of these issues (1991, 160). The dearth of long-term studies of weight loss make it unclear if "obese" people who lower their weights to the so-called ideal actually lower their risk of mortality and morbidity; indeed, so few obese people manage to achieve and maintain their "ideal weights" for any length of time that the question may be unanswerable (see Brownell 1991; Brownell and Wadden 1991; Jarrett 1988). Given these doubts about whether the "ideal weights" often given by the data derived for life insurance actuarial tables really represent the best weights for patients, and especially given the extreme dubiousness of the claim that many, let alone most, "obese" individuals *could* achieve such weights without heroic and possibly dangerous and unhealthy methods, Brownell and Wadden suggest that the concept of a patient's "ideal weight" be replaced by that of a "reasonable weight" for a given patient (1991, 160). A "reasonable weight" takes into account "a client's weight history, social circumstances, metabolic profile, and other factors" such as the health problems that the treatment is designed to deal with (1991, 160–61, 158–59). In general, they suggest that the "goal weight should be no lower than the client's lowest weight which has been maintained for at least a year since age 21," clearly a weight that will often be far above the "ideal weight" given by life insurance tables, and they further note that the weight suggested by this goal will often have to be revised upward (1991, 160–61).

Brownell and Wadden therefore suggest that obesity not be dealt with as a general medical condition requiring treatment to achieve some "nonobese" weight, but rather that "obese" patients be treated on an individualized basis, with treatments focused on existing medical problems or clear precursors to problems (1991, 158–59). For them, "achieving an important health benefit can be used as one index of successful treatment" where some of these health benefits are "less tangible effects such as improved mobility," and that achieving "goal weights," the traditional measure of success, should be at the very most a distant consideration (1991, 159). Similar points are made by Kassirer and Angell (1998). They too recommend that "doctors need to tailor their advice to each patient" and "recommend weight loss if a patient is suffering from health problems that can be ameliorated by weight loss . . . or [is] clearly in jeopardy" but otherwise that doctors should "be cautious about exhorting patients to lose weight" (1998, 53). They warn that "until we have better data bout the risks of being overweight and benefits of trying to lose weight, we should remember that the cure for obesity may be worse than the condition" (1998, 53).

The Medicalization of Preference

Thinking of obesity as a disease, as a problem in and of itself, creates a category of people: the "obese," or the "overweight," or simply the "fat." Thinking in terms of "ideal weights," body mass indexes or body fat percentages problematizes deviations from these "ideals." Even if it should turn out that some relatively low body fat percentage, BMI, or weight, if "achieved" through a naturally low set point and existing in a certain sort of social system, has associated with it significantly lower risks of certain medical problems, this says nothing about at what weight *everyone* should strive to be. The health benefits of having always been thin may not accrue to those who have to struggle to be thin. Nor, obviously, do epi"demiological studies of the relationship between weight and disease illuminate any of the relevant causal pathways between, for example, having a low BMI and having a decreased risk for certain classes of medical problems. However, as long as being over a certain weight, BMI, or body fat percentage is regarded as having a certain medical condition—that is, as defining obesity—and is widely associated with health problems of one sort or another, the meaning of obesity as a negative trait will undoubtedly remain fixed.

Even as the moral status of obesity is thrown into doubt by research implying that it is not in general the result of "choices" made and that it is very difficult to change, its status as a "problem" is strengthened. That is, making obesity out as having a partial genetic etiology does nothing to make it an acceptable, let alone a desirable, body type. Obese people may no longer be explicitly blamed for their condition, but are definitely thought of as having a condition, a condition that, ideally, should be "treated" and, preferably, "cured." So far, however, dieting, behavior modification therapy, drugs, and surgery have failed to consistently bring obese individuals into line with "ideal weights" and keep them there (see for example Brownell and Wadden 1991). Many of these approaches have, however, been blamed for causing serious medical problems themselves (see for example Kassirer and Angell 1998, 52–53).

There was enormous early hope for approaches to treating obesity that took a molecular tack, prompted by the success of researchers in isolating the cause of obesity in certain variants of mice and "treating" them for it. Mice with two mutant copies of a certain gene (the *ob* gene) end up radically obese (see Barinaga 1995; Pelleymounter et al. 1995; Halaas et al. 1995; and Campfield et al. 1995). In 1995 three research teams independently found that the normal product of this gene, dubbed "leptin" by the team led by Friedman (see "Food for Fat Cats," 60–61), when injected into *ob/ob* mice (mice with two copies of the *ob* gene mutation) results in radical weight and body fat loss. Injected into either "wild-type" or ordinarily lean strains, the rats lost significant amounts of weight, and essentially all their body fat (Barinaga, 1995, 475; Pelleymounter et al. 1995, 540, 541, 542; Halaas et al. 1995, 543, 544 545; and Campfield et al. 1995, 546, 547, 548). However, obese mice with a different genetic defect, so-called *db/db* mice, seem to produce relatively large amounts of leptin themselves, and were all but unaffected by even massive doses of the *ob* protein; apparently leptin does not have the ordinary effect on their weight-regulatory systems for one reason or another (a problem with the receptor sites is suspected) (see Halaas et al. 1995, 543, 544; Campfield et al. 1995, 546, 547, 548; "Food for Fat Cats," 60–61). It soon became clear that the effectiveness of leptin for treating human obesity would depend critically on whether human obesity generally results from problems with receptor sites, leptin production, or some other part of the pathway entirely ("Food for Fat Cats," 61; Barinaga 1995, 476). Currently it seems clear that the majority of obese individuals would not be susceptible to leptin as a treatment method, since they already produce much larger than normal amounts of it (see Considine et al. 1996; Maffei et al. 1995). However, it may be the case that, given the heterogeneity and multiple etiologies of human obesity in general, drugs based on leptin will prove effective for some segment of the population with diagnosable obesity (Montague 1997 is suggestive, for example).

The effect of leptin on normal, wild-type mice seems to imply that people *without* obvious weight problems may be among the most natural targets for such a drug (Barinaga 1995, 476; "Food for Fat Cats," 61); while this idea has yet to be tested in humans, the potential for such a drug to be abused has already been noted (Barinaga 1995, 476). If the work on wild-type mice proves to be a good indication, such a drug would allow "normal-weight . . . people to drop pounds without changing" their eating or exercise habits (Barinaga 1995, 476). If such should turn out to be the case, it will be interesting to see how many of the "health benefits" that supposedly accrue to low body fat percentages and low BMIs will accrue to such artificially controlled body fat percentages.

If a drug were developed that permitted maintainable weight loss in a significant portion of people diagnosed as obese, even if it produced no health benefits, there is good reason to suspect that it would be used. And, given the option of having an "ideal" weight, there is every reason to suspect that many people will "choose" to use such a drug to achieve that weight, whether or not such a weight has any health benefits, and indeed, even if it carried with it certain risks. In fact, it is already clear that people are willing to take real risks to shed weight, even when they are not suffering health problems associated with obesity (see Brownell 1991). The "fen-phen" fiasco, where two diet drugs (fenfluramine and phentermine) that had been separately approved for short-term use proved to be quite dangerous when used in combination for long periods, revealed just how many people under "treatment" for obesity with prescription drugs were not in fact clinically obese (see Kolata 1997 for a summary; Connolly et al. 1997). Talk of "controlling" access to leptin notwithstanding, it strikes me as likely that it will be abused, whether legally or illegally, if it should prove to as effective in causing nonobese humans to shed body fat as it has been in ordinary mice.

Drug-based treatments are a real threat, even if they are successful. If they should prove successful, obesity would become fixed not just as a disease, but as a *treatable* disease, whatever the risks and benefits of the treatments. And, under these conditions, there is every reason to think that it would once again be socially unacceptable to be overweight. Being overweight would once again be constructed as a choice, and a choice that people would be expected *not* to make.

The nearly universal, and ill-supported, assumption that obesity is always a medical problem represents the medicalization of what is nothing more than a cultural preference for a certain body type. Recognizing that, except where losing weight is necessary to treat or avoid some specific medical problem, weight and body fat percentages are not necessarily problems requiring medical treatment would be the first step in creating a new approach to "obesity," an approach that treated a wider range of body types as part of the normal range of human phenotypes, rather than as problems to be solved. Such an approach to obesity would recognize that the "ideal weights" given by actuarial tables and population studies are local to the point of being meaningless, and that the heterogeneity of etiologies of high body fat percentages make such numbers useless for predicting medical outcomes in individual cases.

Perhaps, with such an approach, weight could become less of a social concern as well. Indeed, only after this culture's obsession with low body fat percentages is somewhat ameliorated will it be possible to tell how many of the negative effects of being overweight are really negative effects of continual dieting, massive weight cycling, and the psychological stress associated with being "fat" in a culture obsessed with "thin." Indeed, if one feels that a culture that makes a significant percentage of people with weights close to what is really an absurdly low ideal feel that they are *still* "overweight" is deeply problematic, one should be concerned about *any* system that associates being overweight with far more problems than any reasonable interpretation of the evidence would permit (see for example Powers 1988, 33, and Brownell 1991, 3–4). Brownell ends "Dieting and the Search for the Perfect Body" with a quote from Freedman: "You have a right—and a responsibility—to judge yourself according to realistic standards, a right to feel comfortable in your own skin" (Brownell 1991, 10, quoting Freedman 1988). For the medical community to recognize, and work to publicize, that the range of ordinary, normal, and even desirable human body types includes many this culture regards as overweight would be a good first step to realizing such a goal. Working to find new "wonder drugs" that will allow people with perfectly normal body types to achieve body fat percentages in the single digits should be recognized as a distinct step backward.

CHAPTER 9
CONTRACT PREGNANCIES AND GENETIC PARENTHOOD

Parents, Genes, and the Law

The legal decisions surrounding contract pregnancies, often called surrogae mother contracts, have been part of a process of defining parenthood, at least in legal terms, as being *primarily* about *genetic parenthood*. While there have been relatively few cases that directly test this point, those that exist are very suggestive. The rights and responsibilities associated with parenthood in this culture are, more and more often, being associated with being a genetic parent. Such an emphasis on the genetic as defining parenthood is deeply disturbing, in at least several different ways.

In this chapter, my primary concern will be on the way in which a continuing legal emphasis on the genetic as defining parenthood might tend to undermine other more cultural and relationship-based definitions. Insofar as one believes that parenthood is about being in certain sorts of relationships to other people, a series of legal moves that make parenthood out to be strictly a matter of the genetic is particularly worrisome.[1]

This chapter begins with a review of the current legal situation surrounding contract pregnancies, as well as other legal decisions regarding the nature of parenthood of interest to these issues. The trend I trace is toward making the law compatible with an extreme emphasis on the genetic for defining parenthood. While this occasionally takes the form of arguments *from* the genetics being used directly in legal decisions, I argue that even where arguments from the genetic emphasis are not used *explicitly* by the judges and no explicit emphasis on the genetic is stated in the law, the trend toward compatibility with such an emphasis that I trace in this chapter can be read properly as displaying an *implicit* concern with the genetic. The trend toward making parenthood out to be a matter of genetics grows out of the same sort of cultural emphasis on the genetic that makes, for example, such things as major sequencing projects (e.g., the Human Genome Project) look like plausible places to spend public money, and that popularizes those research projects into human genetics that, for example, estimate heritability or work to find genes associated with various complexes. Finally, I argue that a move to the genetic as defining parenthood should be resisted. Some of the cases that have helped move the definition of parenthood toward being strictly a genetic matter have already influenced decisions in other cases, and influenced them in ways that I argue have had the effect of excluding some people from parenthood in ways that I think ought to be regarded as problematic. In the end, I argue that there is an important sense in which genetic parenthood, narrowly construed, should count much less, legally and culturally.

Since my focus is on the way that a cultural emphasis on the genetic inspires a type of reasoning that is particularly problematic when used to define "parenthood," my attention to pregnancy contracts emerges in large part from the way in which they serve as legal test cases in this area, because of the way in which they separate out many of the different possible aspects of "parenthood." While this is a disturbing feature of contract pregnancies, the other ways in which they are disturbing—ways related to the current economic and racial inequalities in the United States, and those related to the gender inequalities and injustices that exist in contemporary society—seem to many people to be clearly more problematic and of a more immediate concern (see for example Satz 1992). My focus on the genetic aspects of these cases should *not* be taken to imply that a system of regulating pregnancy contracts such that they no longer require or inspire a focus on the genetic would make them acceptable within a just society. But I do want to argue that even if those gender and racial problems were ameliorated, the problematic aspects of defining parenthood as being primarily about a genetic relationship would remain.

Legal Parenthood, Contract Pregnancies, and the Genetic Connection

In this section, several different ways of being declared a "parent" (in a legal sense) are discussed. The first legal cases considered are those that surrounded contract pregnancies. In these cases, it is argued that having a genetic relationship to the child in question has been taken to be the deciding factor in several important cases. The next cases considered are those involving artificial insemination by donor (AID) and in vitro fertilization (IVF) with donor eggs. In these cases, it might seem that genetic relationships are deliberately downplayed; however, I argue that properly understood, these cases are still compatible with an emphasis on the genetic, just not necessarily an "absolute" one.

Contract Pregnancies: Ways of Being a Parent

While contract pregnancies have become something of a testing ground for the law's conception of what it is to be a parent, most contract pregnancies, of course, do not result in legal cases. Indeed, in part because of the practice's shaky legal status, most contract pregnancies are never reported in any context where they can be tracked (see Lascarides 1997; Keane 1981; and Corea 1985). This paucity of cases, combined with the long lags resulting from the appeals process, has resulted in the law remaining rather unsettled. The occasional addition of new legislation at the state level and the rewriting of pregnancy contracts to take account of this, followed by a new round of legal cases, also hasn't helped matters. For the most part, then, the conclusions I'll be drawing from looking at the legal cases, and the reasoning that went into those legal decisions made, will be tentative (see also Lascarides 1997 on the "unsettled" nature of law in this arena).

Contract pregnancies actually come in several different forms. In what is currently the most common, the man who is to be the genetic father contracts with a woman who is to be both the genetic and gestational mother. After being impregnated with his sperm (usually, although not always, through artificial insemination) and carrying the child to term, she agrees to terminate all her parental rights at the child's birth (or as soon after the child's birth as the law in whatever state the birth takes place permits).[2] In this form, then, the birth mother is both the genetic and gestational mother, and it is the genetic father with whom she has the contract. While in general both the media at large and the legal and academic communities have used the term "surrogate mother" for the birth mothers in contract pregnancies, and generally referred to the contracts involved as "surrogate motherhood" contracts or agreements, this seems wrongheaded. As Satz 1992 (as well as, for example, Judge Wilentz in the *Baby M* case) correctly points out, the birth mothers in most contract pregnancies are the genetic and gestational mothers of the children in question: in no sense are they "surrogate" (see Satz 1992, 107; Ellman et al. 1991, 1307). Even in the cases discussed below, where the so-called surrogate is the gestational but not genetic mother, the term seems misapplied.

In any event, when the contract pregnancy takes the form of a genetic father contracting with the woman who is to be both the genetic and gestational mother, the contracts are often formed so as to explicitly exclude mention of the genetic father's wife, if there is one, in part to avoid legal prohibitions against baby-selling and adoptions undertaken for financial gain. The laws in question make agreements to surrender children for adoption in exchange for monetary compensation void, but people arguing that contract pregnancies do not violate these laws point out that it is not an adoption in the usual sense that is going on at all. Instead, they claim, there is "merely" a transfer of all rights to one of the parents involved—there is just the termination of all the mother's parental rights, not an adoption at all. Since the adoption proceedings that make the wife of the genetic father the legal mother take place *after* all the terms of the contract have been fulfilled, they are not a part of it.

While courts have differed on whether these contracts avoid prohibitions on baby-selling, in disputes arising from contract pregnancies where the "surrogate" is both the genetic and gestational mother, courts have tended to regard the pregnancy contract as either entirely void or at least as voidable, and have treated the case as more or less a traditional custody battle between the genetic and gestational mother and the genetic father.[3] In cases where the contract pregnancy is undertaken for money, this tends to have the effect of favoring the genetic father, since "best interest" clauses will tend, in general, to support married couples capable of paying on the order of ten thousand dollars, plus attendant medical expenses, over those women or couples whose financial situations are such that they are willing to undergo a pregnancy at least in part for that money (see Corea 1985, 228ff.).

It was in large part this kind of "best interest" reasoning that resulted in Baby M being placed with the Sterns, who were, respectively the genetic father and stepmother. However, Mary Beth Whitehead, the genetic and gestational mother, was eventually granted some visitation rights, in keeping with her role as the legal mother of Baby M. (see *In the Matter of Baby M* or Ellman et al. 1991, 1322 for summary and discussion). While the majority of cases of contract pregnancy are not undertaken primarily, or indeed at all, for monetary gain, a relatively large percentage of those that have been legally contested have certainly had the appearance of having been undertaken at least in large part for monetary gain (see Ellman et al. 1991, 1322–30, esp. 1326; but see Arneson 1992, 154–55). It is likely, though, that most of the contract pregnancy arrangements are between family members, and are made without very much in the way of formal arrangements or contracts at all.

It is interesting to note that until recently the sort of "best interest" reasoning discussed above would have seemed very alien in the context of custody disputes. Until relatively recently, young children's best interest was usually taken to coincide with maternal custody (see Ellman et al. 1991, notes on the "Tender Years Doctrine," 502–3). This, though, has changed in part as laws were rewritten to be phrased in "gender neutral" ways (see Ellman et al. 1991, 508). While women obtain sole custody after divorce in some 90 percent of cases, the vast majority of these are undisputed, and while studies of the results in contested cases give wildly varying results, there is at least not a particularly marked preference for sole maternal custody, and there is perhaps a preference for sole paternal custody. What to make of this, however, remains somewhat unclear (see Ellman et al. 1991, 508–10). Historically in English law, men were assumed to have an "absolute right" to their children and women were almost never granted custody (Corea 1985, 288). (For summaries of some of the legal practices involving best interest clauses, see Ellman et al. 1991, 500ff.).

In the other primary form of contract pregnancies, the genetic and gestational mothers are separated in the following way: the contracting parties use only their own genetic material; the man's sperm and woman's egg are fertilized via in vitro fertilization techniques, and the resulting embryo is then implanted in the womb of a third party, again often awkwardly called the "surrogate mother." In this case, the birth mother (the "surrogate") is the gestational mother, and the contracting parties are the genetic father and genetic mother,[4] respectively.[5] In the vast majority of cases of contract pregnancies involving in vitro fertilization, the man and woman involved in donating genetic material are a married couple; many firms dealing in contract pregnancies require that the contracting man be part of a married couple, and often that his wife be infertile, apparently for reasons of political expedience (see Corea 1985, 217). There have, of course, been exceptions; however, despite the potential, neither technique has yet been made widely available to, for example, same-sex couples (see Hollandsworth 1995).

There has only been one case, *Johnson v. Calvert*, where the so-called surrogate mother was the gestational mother but not the genetic mother, and there was a conflict between the gestational and the genetic mother for custody.[6] Here the legal situation was interpreted rather differently than in those cases where the gestational mother was also the genetic mother; indeed, in this case, the gestational mother was denied all legal rights associated with parenthood. The initial rulings, as well the decision of the appeals court, made explicit reference to the importance of the genetic relationship in framing their decision. Judge Richard Parslow (a trial judge in Orange County, California) ruled that the gestational mother in the case was "analogous to a "foster parent'" and that her womb was merely "the home in which she had sheltered and fed another's child," and, on that reasoning, "granted the genetic parents full parental rights" (see Ellman et al. 1991, 1324; see Superior Court of Orange County, Nos. X-633190 and AD-57638). Indeed, Judge Parslow based his decision explicitly on such things as the high heritability of IQ and other features (op. cit.; see also Krim 1996 for discussion). As this case worked its way to the California Supreme Court, several courts in between reaffirmed the emphasis on the genetic. For example, the court of appeals noted,

> As evidence at trial showed, the whole process of human development is "set in motion by the genes." There is not a single organic system of the human body not influenced by an individual's underlying genetic makeup. Genes determine the way physiological components of the human body, such as the heart, liver, or blood vessels operate. Also, according to the expert testimony received at trial, it is now thought that genes influence tastes, preferences, personality styles, manners of speech and mannerisms. (Cal. Rptr. 286 1991, 381)

However, when the case got to the California Supreme Court, the justices who decided the case thought the situation a bit more complex than the trial court or appellate court decisions would imply. In the majority decision, they noted that each woman in the case had submitted acceptable proof of maternity under California law: in Crispina Calvert's case, blood and genetic testing; and in Anna Johnson's case, proof of having given birth to the child. Further, the justices noted that there is "no clear legislative preference" in civil code for one form of proof over the other (*Johnson v. Calvert* 5 Cal. 4th, 92). Although they approvingly quote Hill's argument that "while gestation may demonstrate maternal status . . . it is possible that the common law viewed genetic consanguinity as the basis for maternal rights" and that "under this interpretation gestation simply would be irrefutable evidence of the more fundamental genetic relationship," apparently they did not follow this reasoning explicitly in formulating their decision (*Johnson v. Calvert*, quoting Hill, 92–93).[7]

The judges in this case decided that there was a definite sense in which either woman, but not both, could be the natural mother. That is to say, the majority decision recognized that under law either woman could be the natural mother, and took as its task deciding *which* woman that would be.

Indeed, several of the justices noted their explicit disapproval for any system that would fail to explicitly choose between the two women. The *Los Angeles Times* quoted Justice Panelli as wondering whether having both "a genetic parent . . . and a gestational parent" could even be a "traditional family unit," and Chief Justice Lucas as observing "that it could prove awkward for a child to grow up with both a 'mother' and a 'genetic progenitor.'" The judges note that while "multiple parent arrangements [are] common in our society," they "decline to accept the contention of amicus curiae the American Civil Liberties Union (ACLU) that we should find the child has two mothers" because they can "see no compelling reason to recognize such a situation here" (Johnson v.Calvert, 92, n. 8).

Given that the judges felt they had to decide between the two putative mothers and that they found that there was no legislative law available to "break the tie," they argued that it is the intentions of the parties involved, as demonstrated in part by the "surrogacy" contract, that should be used to decide parentage. At one point, the majority decision states,

> We conclude that although [the Uniform Parentage Act] recognizes both genetic consanguinity and giving birth as means of establishing a mother and child relationship, when the two means do not coincide in one woman, she who intended to procreate the child—that is, she who intended to bring about the birth of the child that she intended to raise as her own—is the natural mother under California law. (*Johnson v. Calvert, 93*)

In this case, they noted, it was the intentions of Crispina and Mark Calvert that resulted in the existence of the child and hence Crispina Calvert was the "natural mother" under California law.

Indeed, the only dissenting decision, Justice Kennard's, took issue not with having to pick one of two potential mothers, nor even with the particular mother chosen, but rather with the criteria used. Justice Kennard argued that using the parties' intentions as expressed in the "surrogacy contract" risked the "abuse of surrogacy arrangements" and that instead the standard used should be "the best interests of the child" (*Johnson v. Calvert*, 507).[8] While Justice Kennard noted that "pregnancy entails a unique commitment, both physiological and emotional, to an unborn child," he also claims that "no less substantial . . . is the contribution of the woman from whose egg the child developed and without whose desire the child would not exist" (*Johnson v. Calvert*, 506).

So, while in the end the California Supreme Court did not entirely discount the role of the gestational in its majority decision, it did deny

Johnson all parental rights, in large part because of the Calverts' genetic relationship. In 1993 the United States Supreme Court declined to review the case, letting those decisions affirming Parslow's original decision stand (see *Johnson v. Calvert* 510 U.S. 874).

An Ohio court found itself ruling on a case with superficially similar facts (*Belsito et al. v. Clark et al.*). In this case, however, there was no conflict between any of the parties. The gestational mother (Carol Clark) was more than willing to give up the child she was carrying to term, and the genetic parents (Anthony and Shelly Belsito) more than willing to assume all the rights and responsibilities of parenthood.[9] The only issue turned out to be a local hospital's unwillingness to list Shelly Belsito as the mother on the birth certificate (*Belsito v. Clark*, 67 Ohio Misc. 2d, 58); the court action was a request to have the Belsitos declared the legal parents. In this case, the court ruled in no uncertain terms that "the law requires that, because Shelly Belsito and Anthony Belsito provided the child with its genetics, they must be designated as the legal and natural parents" (58). The ruling continued:

> . . . there is abundant precedent for using the genetics test for identifying a natural parent. . . . The genetic parent can guide the child from experience through the strengths and weaknesses of a common ancestry of genetic traits . . . [the genetic test] should remain the primary test for determining the natural parent, or parents, in nongenetic-providing surrogacy cases. (64)

Indeed, in *Belsito v. Clark* the court was not at all sympathetic to the "intent" doctrine put forward in *Johnson v. Calvert* and *McDonald v. McDonald* (see below). Here, the argument was given that "intent to procreate" is difficult to prove, does not take sufficient account of public policy considerations, and fails "to fully recognize the genetic provider as having the right to choose or to consent" (*Belsito v. Clark*, 63). The court notes that the "procreation of a child, that is, the replication of the unique genes of an individual, should occur only with the consent of that individual" (64). In other words, the provider of the genetic material for a pregnancy can only lose his or her rights if explicit consent is given (as in "egg donation" cases, such as *McDonald v. McDonald*, below); the gestational mother, however, apparently has no such presumption of rights.[10]

The Mysteries of Artificial Insemination by Donor and In Vitro Fertilization with Donor Eggs: Finding a Parent in the Absence of Genetic Relationships
While the reasoning alluded to above is far from being universally accepted, the fact that such arguments can get made at all suggests at least

a certain emphasis on the genetic over other ways of defining parenthood. And it is at least in part because such arguments do get made that Satz, for example, worries that if "[g]enes alone are taken to define natural and biological motherhood"; that is, if "women's rights and contributions [are defined] in terms of those of men," courts will "fail to recognize an adequate basis for women's rights and needs" (1992, 127–28). While this reasoning is made obvious in cases of contract pregnancies, it is of course applicable in cases of "ordinary" pregnancies as well, and its extension to ordinary cases is, as noted above, at least equally worrisome.

Artificial insemination by donor (AID) cases, however, might seem to point in the opposite direction. In these cases, in a procedure that is medically indistinguishable from that used in contract pregnancies where the woman is both the genetic and gestational mother, a woman is impregnated by artificial insemination. In most cases, it is the wife of an infertile man who is impregnated by the sperm of a donor, usually unknown to the parties involved. In these cases, the law treats her consenting husband as the father of the resulting child, despite his lack of any genetic relationship to the child.[11] If there is, as I am claiming, some tendency for various court decisions to point toward at least a general compatibility with a genetic emphasis, AID cases are clearly problematic for that position.

Or so it might seem. One key feature of most AID cases, suggested above, is the anonymity of the sperm donor. Sperm are taken from the donor, waivers signed, and the sperm then used without the donor's knowledge (see Corea 1985, 53–55). Often the records are destroyed, at least in part to ensure that there will be no future conflicts (Corea 1985, 54). This de facto prevents any conflicts from arising, as there is no other father, especially no genetic father, to claim the rights associated with parenthood. However, in cases where for one reason or another a sperm donor *can* identify the resulting child as being (genetically) his, courts have been much more willing to consider his rights. Ellman et al. 1991 cite the following case (a lower-court decision on this case is also alluded to in Corea 1985, 49ff.). In *Jhordan C. v. Mary K.* (see 179 Cal. Appl 3d386, 224 Cal. Rptr. 530 [1986]) the sperm donor brought action to establish paternity and visitation rights, and won, although the mother retained sole custody. The court found that the statute excluding any paternity rights for sperm donors was inapplicable to AID not performed by a physician (Ellman et al. 1991, 935–36; see also Henry 1993).

I know of no cases where an egg donor has tried to get parental rights. This may be because anonymity is always maintained, as the procedure is nearly impossible to perform outside established medical facilities. In the California Supreme Court's majority decision in the *Johnson v. Calvert* case, however, they suggest that under their analysis in "a true 'egg donation' situation, where a woman gestates and gives birth to a child formed from the egg of another woman with the intent to raise the child as her own, the birth mother is the natural mother under California law," since it is intent that "breaks the tie" between putative mothers (*Johnson v. Calvert* 19 Ca. Rptr., 2d, 93, n. 10). The justices make clear in *Johnson v. Calvert* that it is by analogy to a "true" sperm donor situation, where it is performed by a "licensed physician" and thus anonymity is maintained, that the egg donor situation has the status they think it does (19 California Reporter, 2d, 101). This was the reasoning used in *McDonald v. McDonald*, one of the only legal cases in which egg donation was a relevant factor. Here the gestational mother was impregnated via IVF in a "true" egg donor situation, and, in a postdivorce custody battle, the genetic father claimed that his former wife, the gestational mother of the child, was not a "natural" mother and hence that he should get sole custody. This contention was rebuffed, the court finding that in "a true 'egg donation' situation, where a woman gestates and gives birth to a child formed from the egg of another woman with the intent to raise the child of her own, the birth mother must be deemed the natural mother" (McDonald v. McDonald, 196 A.D.2d 7). One imagines that in an "egg donor" situation performed outside the traditional medical community the situation might be parallel to that of the AID cases where the genetic fathers have managed to win rights. In the absence of such cases, though, the situations must remain unclear.

In any event, recent decisions have tended to be against those laws that create assumptions about parenthood *not* based on genetic relationships. For example, until relatively recently a child born in wedlock was legally assumed to be the legitimate child of the couple involved, and attempts by other men to claim paternity were summarily rebuffed. The laws in these cases, presumption of legitimacy laws, usually stated that the presumption of legitimacy could only be rebutted by the husband or wife, and then only in certain limited circumstances (see Ellman et al. 1991, 937ff. for a summary of some of these cases and for a brief discussion of some of the history and issues involved). Relatively recently, however, this has changed. Recent cases and legislature recognize the legal claims of putative fathers even in cases where the woman involved is married to another man and both she and her husband accept the child as legitimate.[12] Indeed, a California court wrote into its judgment in a "traditional surrogacy" case that the Uniform Parentage Act was inapplicable in this case as "genetic parenthood established by blood tests trumps a presumption based on the cohabitation of a married couple" (*In Re Marriage of Cynthia J.*, 25 Cal. App. 4th, 1225).

There is, then, a growing tendency to take genetic contribution very seriously in deciding issues involving parenthood. Indeed, attention to the details of AID cases reveal them as not nearly as anomalous as might have been thought, and the recent decisions in favor of genetic fathers against presumed fathers—or for that matter in favor of genetic mothers against presumed mothers (see *In Re Marriage of Cynthia J.*, 1225)—follow this trend. Given this, the somewhat tentative conclusions drawn about the reasoning in *Johnson v. Calvert* and *Belsito v. Clark*—that is, that there is a growing tendency for the legal decisions that get made in these cases to be compatible with parenthood being defined in terms of genetic contribution—stand on somewhat firmer ground. While there has not yet been a sweeping decision to treat parenthood as only a genetic phenomenon, that there has been some tendency to move in such a direction seems clear.

In a sense, this follows neatly from a cultural tradition of thinking of biological parenthood as the only parenthood that really matters. Many health insurance policies will cover the often exceedingly high costs of infertility treatments but not the costs of adoption. Bartholet, for example, notes as well the many more subtle ways that society—and more importantly, law—expresses an implicit approval of biological, and an implicit disapproval of adoptive, parenthood (see Bartholet 1993, 34).

The Centrality of the Gene in Pregnancy

There is at least one perspective from which defining parenthood in terms of genetic contribution would seem nonproblematic. Indeed, reading the papers that, for example, many of those people working on human genetics research have published for popular consumption, one might wonder what took the courts so long. Recall the bold claims made by researchers quoted in chapter 2, for example, such as Gilbert's claims that DNA is "the most fundamental property of the body," that the sequence is "what makes us human," and that "how . . . we differ from one another" is a question to be answered by biologists specializing in population genetics (Gilbert 1992, 83–84). Researchers like Hood refer to the genome as "our blueprint for life" and the Human Genome Project as creating "an encyclopedia of life" (1992, 136). Hamer and Copeland's *Living with Our Genes* (1998) is subtitled *Why They Matter More Than You Think*. Given claims and descriptions like these about the importance of the genetic (see chapters 2 and 3 for more examples), an emphasis on the genetic in determining parenthood might seem entirely reasonable. It would be, after all, simply a fact that genetic mothers contributed to the "most fundamental property" of their offspring, while "mere" gestational mothers did not.[13]

Indeed, the way that contract pregnancies are handled by those corporations and individuals who deal in them reveals this sort of genetic emphasis as well. Where the "surrogate" mother is both the genetic and gestational mother, many organizations involved in finding surrogates permit the potential genetic fathers wide latitude in selecting women with the proper set of presumably heritable traits. Keane, an attorney specializing in contract pregnancies and one of the biggest advocates for them, permits selection on such criteria as height, weight, ethnicity, eye color, hair color, complexion, IQ, religion (!), and the like (see Keane 1981, 274, 282ff.; and Corea 1985, 218–19). While it is certainly true that we permit many personal decisions to be made on such bases, keep in mind that in general we do *not* permit people to make, for example, hiring decisions on such bases. Insofar as the surrogate is supposed to be merely an employee producing a product, that such criteria are regarded as permissible and indeed *indispensable*, is deeply problematic. Since some other sort of relationship, one more personal than that of simply producing a product, is hinted at by the permissibility and indispensability of these criteria, we should be disturbed by the desire to construe the relationship, in every other context, in simple commodified terms.

Where the "surrogate" is to be the gestational but not the genetic mother, much less care is taken with regard to the mother's traits (it is worth recalling here that Anna Johnson, the gestational surrogate in *Johnson v. Calvert*, was black, the Calverts white and Filipina). Corea notes that Stephura, who is involved in the contract pregnancy industry, thinks that costs in "surrogacy agreements" will come down in part because once contract pregnancies involve the use of the surrogate only as the gestational mother, "clients will find the breeder's IQ and skin color immaterial" and "surrogate firms" will be able to use women from, for example, Third World countries (Corea 1985, 214–15).

However, for all the emphasis on the genetic, it is important to keep in mind that the sorts of claims about the centrality of the gene cited above as emerging from people involved in certain sorts of human genetics research do not, in fact, emerge from the research as *results;* rather, their status is more that of metaphors. These metaphors provide a guide to both how to pursue research projects in human genetics and how to interpret any results obtained from such research projects (see chapter 2 on the interpretations of claims like these as "methodological" and "causal"). There is, quite obviously, no research that could *show* that, for example, DNA is "the most fundamental property of the body," nor even that the genome is a "blueprint for life." More importantly, the near ubiquity of such claims in the literature should not be taken to imply that they are particularly good metaphors. If the analysis given in the previous chapters is correct about the current state of human genetics research into the etiologies of the variations in complex traits that exist in society, it seems that doubt could easily be cast on any claim that the "genetic" is "central" in any but the most symbolic way.[14]

The Centrality of the Gene to Parenthood Problematized

However, one might still wonder, just why should we care about how parenthood is defined? The cases of legal disputes involving contract pregnancies are rare, and the decisions are nonsystematic enough that, one might argue, it doesn't look like any particular *harm* is done by the occasional stressing of genes. It is suspicious, perhaps, that in all the legal disputes between genetic and gestational mothers, genetic mothers have won. But two cases, it might be argued, hardly demonstrate a compelling trend. However, these decisions do not just form precedents for the relatively rare legal decisions that are identical; rather they are used, and used in important ways, in other kinds of cases, and more generally. Explicitly they are used in deciding other legal cases and in formulating policy; implicitly they have the effect of changing conceptions of parenthood in ways that influence (perhaps subtly) other policy issues. Here, after displaying and describing some of these effects, I argue that there is no good reason to accept the trend toward defining parenthood as being primarily about a genetic relationship.

The Legal Influence
How do these relatively rare cases get used? Judge Spicer, the judge in *Belsito v. Clark*, did note that "the legal status of a nongenetic-providing surrogate who claims parental rights is not at issue" in this case, and hence that "this court cannot properly rule upon the issues involved in determining that status" (*Belsito v. Clark*, 67 Ohio Misc. 2d, 65).[15] So there was, we might have thought, no danger of the case being used to determine custody issues where there *was* a conflict. However, this is not to say that Judge Spicer was unaware that his decision could be setting a precedent, merely that deciding whether the "natural parent" should always be the "legal" parent was not at issue here. Indeed, Pierce-Gealy quotes Judge Spicer as saying (in interviews) that while the case was "common sense" he still tried to formulate his decision carefully:

> I've learned that you have to look at the rule you're setting out to see if it is a good rule for a variety of cases. (1995, 538, n. 28)

How, then, has this case been used? The only case in which it appears to have been used in directing the decision is that of *Liston v. Pyles* (No. 97APF01-137, 1997 Ohio App. Lexis 3627). Not surprisingly, the case raises issues of legal parenthood. In this case, Tamara Pyles and Marla Liston, who had been in a relationship for over fifteen years, decided to raise a child together, and decided that Pyles would be the biological mother. Three years after the birth of the child, Connor, the relationship ended. Liston brought legal action against Pyles, desiring that she be granted visitation rights and shared parenting responsibilities (Lexis 3627, 1–2). The court found, with the trial court, that since Liston was not a "natural" parent, as defined in *Belsito v. Clark*, and had never formally adopted the child, she was in no way a "parent" and had no legal rights nor responsibilities with respect to Connor (Lexis 3627, 8).

There is another way to view this case, however, which the one dissenting judge, Judge Tyack, took. He argued that the "facts before us indicate that Connor was indeed the appellant's child as well as the appellee's" (Lexis 3627, 32). His reasoning was as follows:

> The facts in the record before us indicate appellant was actively involved in the decision to bear this child. Appellant nurtured this child and provided for this child's well-being. . . . This was a sixteen-year, committed relationship between two people that resulted in the birth of a child. . . . The birth was a planned one, the purpose of which was to extend an already existing family unit. After the birth, the child was cared for by both parties. Wills and a trust fund were modified and/or formed by both parties to provide for the new addition to their family. (Lexis 3627, 37)

For Judge Tyack, being a parent was not a matter of being in a certain *genetic* relationship with a child, but a certain *social* relationship. And the majority opinion's concentration on the genetic, Tyack implied, had the effect of denying the importance of that social relationship.

It is, of course, unclear whether the majority opinion of the court was actually influenced by *Belsito v. Clark*, or whether the judges were simply seizing upon a convenient precedent. Certainly, many courts have been reluctant to acknowledge the rights of homosexual parents, and it is certainly imaginable that the court's real difficulty in this case was in seeing an openly lesbian woman as a potential parent (see Hollandsworth 1995; Ellman et al. 1991, 517–23). But even if this was the case in *Liston v. Pyles*, being able to cite *Belsito v. Clark* allowed them to hide behind a definition of "parenthood" rather than having to confront what may have otherwise looked like an antihomosexual bias. And while such a bias in law and lower courts has been upheld on appeal to higher courts (see Ellman et al. 1991, 517–23; Hollandsworth 1995), having to confront it openly presents at least the possibility of objecting to it. As it stands, the stress on the "genetic" aspects of being a parent can be used to make certain kinds of parents look like nonparents to a court.

Ways of Being a Parent, Revisited
There are currently many ways of being a parent that are recognized by at least some courts and some civil codes. One can be a "natural" mother at the very least by giving birth to the child, being the source of the child's genetics (half, the "egg" half), or "causing" the child to be born and "intending" to raise the child. One can be a "natural" father through at least "intent" and being the source of the child's genetics (half, the "sperm" half). All of these "ways" of being a parent can be pulled apart by contemporary reproductive technologies.[16]

Most commonly, of course, far from being deliberately pulled apart, all the ways of being a "natural" parent converge. And to ask in the cases where there is a total convergence which aspects are the most important is probably perverse; attempting to figure why exactly the genetic and gestational mother of a planned child who has also raised that child for several years is a "natural" mother strikes me as a senseless endeavor. The question is what to do in cases where these different ways of being a parent fail to converge, and in those cases looking toward the more normal cases may actually be an error.

Because while, for example, genetic parenthood is a part of "normal" cases, I believe it is in fact the least satisfactory way of dealing with divergent cases. Indeed, modern reproductive technologies are pulling the genetic ever further from the other aspects of parenthood. In the case of traditional AID, considering it a "treatment" for male infertility is obviously ludicrous (see Corea 1985, 53ff.). However, actual sperm transplants would make a more plausible "cure" for male infertility (see Brinster, and Zimmerman, 1994). While, should this technology be used on humans, it would still not result in the man's own DNA being replicated, the sperm would be formed within his own body—they would just not be based on his own DNA. Ovary transplants have long been used in experimental animals, and the situation if used in humans would be nearly parallel (see Plomin et al. 1990, 272–74). In these cases, to think that "natural" parenthood still resided with the genetic would be absurd. A sperm donor whose sperm were used to refertilize another man should, it seems plain, have no

parental rights or responsibilities toward those children the newly fertilized man fathers in what would seem a perfectly ordinary way. Similarly, a
woman with transplanted ovaries who conceives, gestates, and gives birth
to a child in otherwise ordinary circumstances would clearly be as "natural" a mother as any.

While genetic- and phenotypic-level relationships are often cited as
reasons why genetic parenthood should, in one way or another, "count,"
even in hypothetical cases like the above, the arguments for this range
from weak to bizarre. One claim often heard is that one should know who
one's genetic parents are because of, for example, the threat of genetic disease (see for example Koehler 1996; Behne 1996–97; Weiss 1997).
Whatever the force or plausibility of this argument, it is clearly *not* an
argument for granting parental rights and responsibilities on the basis of
the genetic, but rather just what it claims to be prima facie—at best an
argument for knowing who one's genetic parents are for medical, not
social, reasons. Occasionally, phenotypic correlations are cited as a reason
genetic parenthood should matter; this, it seems to me, comes down to
the fact that some children look something like their genetic parents (see
Hill 1991, 371). Why this is any reason at all for genetic parents to have
rights or responsibilities remains, to me, entirely mysterious. That two
people look similar is not a reason for granting rights or responsibilities in
any other legal cases, and certainly, if not for the causal aspect of parenthood, thinking that someone was a natural parent because they happened
to *look* like the child would be crazy. More prosaically, while little is yet
known about its effects broadly, clearly that the gestational environment
is also quite important in terms of phenotypic similarities and differences,
and in some cases research has hinted that it is much more important than
the genetic relationships (see Cropanzano and James 1990, 435). Even if
causal roots of phenotypic similarities matter, which seems implausible,
they do not point unequivocally toward the genetic.

The questions of who is a "natural" parent and who should get the legal
and social rights and responsibilities associated with parenthood cannot
be considered apart from the situation in which the question arises. In the
case of, for example, traditional paternity suits, the issue is primarily one
of financial obligation. In the United States, it was generally the case, at
least until relatively recently, that an unmarried man could escape paternity suits by claiming either not to have had sexual relations with the
woman in question during the relevant period, or by giving evidence that
another man had also done so (the so-called *exceptio plurium concubuenium*
defense). In many countries, though, the *exceptio plurium* defense has

never been allowed (see Ellman et al. 1991, 891–94) and, indeed, the law in Denmark imposed "an obligation of support upon all of the men who had intercourse with the woman during the relevant time" (Ellman et al. 1991, 894; see also Logdberg 1978).

One possible view is that such a system, if more widely adopted, would have the advantage of treating the relationship between the woman involved and the man as key, and put less emphasis on the chance occurrences that govern the outcome. It is also possible that such a system, properly enforced, would be a boon to child welfare, at least in *financial* terms. The California Supreme Court's reluctance to even consider the possibility that a child might have multiple "natural" mothers makes reform in such a direction quite unlikely, however. But it is still imaginable that in at least some paternity cases, the issue of whether a man should have to, for example, pay child support might not be best viewed as a matter of genetic relationships at all. Another view might find that looking toward other sorts of relationships, such as the sexual relationship, would be a more reasonable start. In fact, even in the United States some "modern courts occasionally permit juries to find defendants liable despite serological evidence of nonpaternity" (Ellman et al. 1991, 894). This is at least evidence that a more widespread system of looking back toward personal and social relationships rather than to "causal" happenstance would not be rejected as completely absurd in the context of the current legal system of the United States. Under this interpretation, Hill's analysis, as used in *Johnson v. Calvert*, is entirely backward—it is not that the gestational is a proxy for the "more fundamental" genetic relationship at all; rather, the genetic can be a proxy for establishing a "more fundamental" relationship between the putative parents.

As a cross-cultural aside, the reported experiences of the Trobriand Islanders is interesting in this context. Malinowski claimed that they saw no biological connection between children and (living) men (see Malinowski 1916, 221). Whatever we choose to make of claims like these,[17] Malinowski presents compelling evidence that among those islanders he studied, "fatherhood" was about the relationship that the man has to the woman who gives birth to the children. Aside from several incidents where men returned after years of absence and accepted children just born as their own (with all the appropriate joy at having a child) (1916, 223–24), his informants were quite clear that the *only* way a child could be "illegitimate" was by being born to an unwed woman (1916, 222). There is, it should be clear, nothing necessary about the views of parenthood *this* culture has adopted or may yet adopt in the future.

Observations and Conclusions: Against Easy Answers

How these considerations should apply to cases of contract pregnancies, and disputes about parental rights and responsibilities more generally, is not obvious, except that genetic relationships should not be regarded as being the sine qua non of parenthood when making decisions about the distribution of paternal rights and responsibilities. However, it seems equally clear that none of the other considerations, including intent, "causal responsibility" (however construed), and the child's best interests, should be the ultimate arbiter in these cases either. There are problems establishing "intent" in the best of circumstances, and a lack of intent has never been considered a reason for losing parental rights and responsibilities in other cases; similar arguments speak against an argument from some privileged "causal" pathway to parental rights. And there are times when issues like fairness and social justice may well point away from basing decisions on the best interest of children involved (narrowly construed, at least).[18] Rather, these different factors, including the very real relationship at least some gestational mothers develop with the child they give birth to, should be weighed carefully, without any of the different factors being given an absolute priority.

So far, the more or less unique situations that have surrounded each contract pregnancy that has resulted in a legal case have made any general judgments about the way such cases should be treated difficult and, in all likelihood, dangerous. The attention to the genetic has in part emerged from a social climate in which the genetic is given a particularly robust sort of importance, but also in part from a desperation about how else to deal with these cases. The understandable desire to be able to pick out a single criterion for "parenthood" has the unfortunate consequence of pointing in the direction of the genetic; it is the one criterion that would result in there being exactly one father and exactly one mother in every case (at least given current technological limitations; see note 16 above).

However, the value of this desideratum should not be overestimated. Despite the contentions of Justices Panelli and Lucas in *Johnson v. Calvert* that finding some one person to have all the rights and responsibilities of a mother (and by extension, a single person to have all the rights and responsibilities of a father) was of absolutely vital importance, as they also admitted that multiple parenting arrangements are common in this society, it is fair to doubt just how vital maintaining the singularity of such relationships could be. That children clearly need *some* secure relationships with caretakers in their lives is not enough to reach the conclusion that there must be exactly one mother and one father. In some circumstances, children's interests in having secure relationships with caretakers may best be served by other arrangements (multiple parenting arrangements, single parents, etc.). That is to say, while it *is* undeniably vital that children be put in relationships with adults that will be secure, long-term, and so on, it is *not* vital that these be any particular *sort* of relationship (i.e., contra the court's decision, it is not vital that there be exactly one mother and exactly one father). And whatever value picking out some one individual to be *the* mother or *the* father may have, it should be clear that there is no one privileged way of doing so that makes sense, either historically or, more broadly, conceptually.

Rather than embrace simplistic and dangerous answers out of desperation, we should embrace the plurality and confusion of such cases, recognizing that different situations call for different solutions and legal decisions. Sometimes, contra Judges Panelli and Lucas, multiple parenting relationships may prove best for everyone concerned (perhaps especially for the children involved); at other times, an attention to children's welfare will require that some individuals be excluded from having the rights and responsibilities of parenthood. Indeed, in some cases it may even turn out that an attention to the genetic will prove important in making decisions. I suspect, however, that, properly conceived, these cases will turn out to be quite a bit rarer than contemporary discourse and legal theory would seem to imply.

CHAPTER 10
THE CONCEPT OF THE ENVIRONMENT

The Environment and the Status Quo

In those projects that attempt to explain variations in complex human traits on the basis of human genetics research, the concept of the environment almost invariably gets used in ways that are conservative. Many of these research projects give the current environment a priority that is hard to defend by, for example, not explicitly exploring the role that the environment, and especially culture, plays in the formation and expression of such traits, and by all too often ignoring the role that, for example, behaviors themselves play in shaping the environment in which genetic effects are supposed to play out in human populations. In many of these research projects, it is the status quo that is the standard against which genetic influences are measured and the effects of intervention are judged. Decisions from what counts as a phenotype worthy of study to what sorts of conditions represent problems worthy of medical intervention are made with respect to contemporary standards, often in an uncritical way. It is in part this unself-critical acceptance of the current environment, and especially the current culture, that so often makes the concept of the environment used in many aspects of human genetics research, and, to a lesser extent, evolutionary theory more broadly, so conservative, in at least its effects, whatever its intentions.

In the previous chapters, a running criticism of the design of research projects in human behavior genetics and related fields, as well as the reporting of the results of such studies, was that they underestimated the possible importance of, and overestimated the likely stability of, the environment, and especially the environment's social aspects. The widespread use of heritability estimates, which are conceptually limited to given populations within given environments, is a prime example (some of these uses were discussed in the previous six chapters). In the cases of the studies that have tried to isolate genes associated with, for example, mood-affective disorders, homosexuality, and violence and criminality, the discounting of the environment, as well as other contexts relevant to understanding what genes "do" in a developmentally relevant sense, was also clear. This discounting has the effect of making the genetics seem much more deterministic and useful than may be the case, and also makes the environment out to be much more unchangeable than many views of current society would admit.

Here I examine the reasons for this discounting, and try to articulate the concept of the environment these studies must be working with if their research is to be interpretable as being useful, or indeed as making sense. I will focus on the relationship between the sort of research that gets done and the way the environment, and especially the social environment, is conceived of. Alternate ways of thinking of the environment, and especially of the relationship organisms have with their environments, will be explored with an eye toward further revealing the inadequacy of the more traditional accounts.

Environment, Organism, and the Modern Synthesis

Odling-Smee, in his "Niche-Constructing Phenotypes" (1988), notes that the modern synthesis, which permitted the "synthesis" of Mendelian genetics with Darwinian evolution, had the important side effect that "autonomous events in the environment" were held "to be exclusively responsible for directing the course of evolution down nonrandom paths" (Odling-Smee 1988, 75; see also Pigliucci and Schlichting 1997). That is, the evolution of organisms was conceived of as caused by environmental events that were thought of as independent of them. The reason for this was that the reconciliation of Mendelian genetics and Darwinian natural selection required that certain "simplifying assumptions" be made:

> First, it was assumed that all heritable traits are determined by genes. Second, it was assumed that natural selection is the only modifying force capable of selecting among different randomly arising, and heritable traits nonrandomly. Third, it was assumed that the environment, including both its biotic and nonbiotic components, is the sole source of natural selection. (Odling-Smee 1988, 74–75)

The strict separation of organisms from their environment is encouraged, although not demanded, by the conceptual framework set up by these assumptions (Odling-Smee 1988, 75).

This separation can be seen in the way evolution by natural selection is traditionally thought of. Levins and Lewontin claim that in modern evolutionary theory the organism is "the object . . . of external forces, which are . . . autonomous and alienated from the organism as a whole" (1985, 87). The idea behind natural selection is, as Lewontin puts it, that the external world "sets certain 'problems' that organisms need to 'solve,'" and "evolution by natural selection is the mechanism for creating these solutions" (1978, 213). "The concept of adaptation," Lewontin notes, "implies a preexisting world that poses a problem to which adaption is the solution" (213).

It is not that this view demands that organisms be thought of as never modifying their environments in ways that affect their reproductive success. Rather, since changes in the environment, even when they are a direct effect of the organism being studied, are able to be decoupled from those organisms' life histories in at least a mathematical sense, one function can be used to describe the evolutionary changes in a species with respect to the environment, and another, quite separate one, to describe changes to the environment—even those changes to the environment that the organisms are themselves causing (see Odling-Smee 1988, 77 and Levins and Lewontin 1985, 104–5).

Odling-Smee notes that the primary attraction of this approach is its simplicity; the evolution of organisms can be described simply as a function of their environments (1988, 75). Since it is assumed that organisms are acted on by their environment and that the environment is describable independent of the organisms in question, other organisms in the same environment can also be treated autonomously. This allows the evolution of organisms, and indeed, even very sophisticated ecosystems, to be modelable in mathematically tractable systems.

These techniques, however, reinforce a habit of thought that makes organisms seem quite separate from their environments. Since changes in gene frequencies are held to be a function of environmental changes, the two are only related insofar as they are functions of each other, even when it is the organisms under consideration themselves that are changing their environment, and even when they are doing so in ways important to their reproductive success. While the mathematical separation of organism and environment does not *demand* the assumption that the organisms in question will be made out to be merely acted upon by an environment entirely outside their control, there is a temptation to read some kind of asymmetrical relationship of this sort into systems where that kind of strict separation is being assumed, even if it assumed only for the purposes of modeling the populations in question.

One way to see how this sort of temptation plays out in practice is to note that the only way the effect organisms have on their environment can be modeled on this system is "self-referentially"; that is, by the change their behaviors have on their genetic fitness (Odling-Smee 1988, 75; for an extended discussion of genetic fitness and different concepts of adaptedness, see Brandon 1990). It is for this reason that Levins and Lewontin object that this approach can make the organism itself out to be irrelevant in an evolutionary sense. Since the only way the organism's modifications of its environment can be modeled is through the effect those modifications have on the organism's fitness, the organism can still be thought of as the passive receiver of environmental forces, even when its own behaviors are changing those forces. And it is this kind of view of the organism as a passive receiver of the forces of environmental selection that makes a view of the organism as nothing more than a way of producing more genes seem at all plausible, since it is only changes in gene frequencies that end up mattering on this view (Levins and Lewontin 1985, 88; see also Plotkin 1988, 10–11). Even those changes in environments directly attributable to the actions of the organisms in question tend to be ignored, or at least their importance radically discounted, on these accounts.

Behavioral Genetics and the Conservative Environment

Contemporary studies of the relationship between genetic variation and variations in complex human traits have been forced to embrace not only those habits of thought that grow out of the modern synthesis, but also assumptions about the relative stability of the environment, or equally strong assumptions about the likely effects of environmental change on the phenotypes in question. Not only must much of the work in the genetics of complex human traits assume that humans are the passive receivers of environmental effects, but, if its techniques are to be thought of as generating any meaningful data at all, the environment must be regarded as broadly stable. It is in part that the formal techniques necessary to model changes in gene frequencies encourage researchers to think of organisms as separate from their environments. Similarly, making use of techniques that estimate broad-sense heritability encourages researchers to make those assumptions that would make those estimates meaningful.

But heritability estimates are about populations with a given genetic distribution within a given set of environmental distributions (see chapter

3). So when an estimate of broad-sense heritability is reported, it can only be assumed to hold within the population studied and in the given environment in which that population existed. More specifically, given a population with a certain distribution of genotypes, an estimate of broad-sense heritability made within that population only holds, in general, for the particular distributions of genotypes across environments present in that population. Even if the environments and genetic populations remain unchanged, changing which genotypes occur with what frequency in which environments can radically change estimates of heritability. This is not at all a trivial point, given many organisms', and perhaps especially humans', ability to choose environments and the way this ability is often ignored in studies of heritability.

Given these problems with the way broad-sense heritability can change within a population, unless some auxiliary assumptions about either the way the trait responds to environmental changes or about the nature of the environment in question itself are made, it is hard to see why estimates of broad-sense heritability would be of interest. For many, indeed for the vast majority of the traits studied in human behavior genetics, we have as yet very little or no evidence about the way the various possible genotypes in question interact with environmental variation with respect to the phenotypic traits under consideration, and so the assumption that they will all respond in an additive fashion might well strike us as at least rather too bold, if not indeed improbable (see chapters 3 and 4). Further, most of what little evidence we do have about the effects of, for example, environmental variation on IQ is about how awful environments, such as those that are massively toxic or nutritionally deprived, influence the traits in question, not about how the trait responds to more "ordinary" variations in environment. Below I argue that the assumption that the environment in which the study took place is at least relatively stable is also deeply problematic.

Other ways in which a faith in the unchanging nature of the current environment slips into behavioral genetics studies include the uncritical acceptance of current standards of behavior, both in picking out which traits to study and in reporting the results from such studies.[1] Given, for example, the contingency of this culture's concepts of sexuality, and the way in which the cultural organization of sexuality seems to influence the behavior of the participants (see chapter 6), the results of studies of the heritability of homosexuality in this culture must be contingent in at least the same way. Doing such studies, then, presupposes that the categories of analysis will remain relevant, and as such, implicitly supports them. That is, if one objects to the categories of analysis, or indeed has doubts about their utility, studying the heritability of traits dependent upon such categories seems at best a bizarre move. Or again, as we saw in chapter 4, part of the argument about interpreting the results on the heritability of learning ability in rats generated by Henderson and those generated by Cooper and Zubek might well come down to what exactly is *meant* by learning ability—what sort of behaviors we choose to count as being an essential part of learning ability. Are variations in motivation and curiosity problems to be eliminated, as Henderson believed, or are they parts of essential components of learning? The way we choose to divide up the world of human traits and variations matters to what sorts of traits, what kinds of behaviors, for example, will turn out to be "heritable"; but it is also a matter of social and political concern, and to support the current ways of dividing up the world is not being neutral but is often to take a stand on these issues.[2]

Policy decisions can be and are influenced by these kinds of background assumptions. In the cases of studies of the genetic bases of mood-affective disorders and criminality and violence, the sorts of decisions that would emerge very naturally from an attention to the genetics would be quite at odds with those that would emerge from a more environment-oriented approach. Again, even if, as claimed, the percentage of crimes committed by criminals with biological problems is over 50 percent, the difference in crime rates between the worst cites in the United States and best cities in Europe is so much greater than that 50 percent that the attempt to reduce crime through biological means should seem totally wrongheaded. In this case it seems we have some evidence, and it points away from a narrow attention to the genetic. On the other hand, we have much less evidence one way or the other for the causes of mood-affective disorders. But if current society is structured such that many people will be unable to live satisfying lives and garner the social rewards necessary to avoid depression, then "curing" them by medically modifying their temperaments, rather than working to create a society in which more people can lead meaningful and rewarding lives, should, I think, seem perverse.

And yet attention to the results of studies in behavioral genetics make medical intervention at the individual level seem much more natural than attempting to change the environment (for example, by changing society). If the given environment is not taken for granted or the phenotype in question not assumed to be insensitive to environmental change in one way or another, the techniques used by the studies become pointless, at least for making predictions or giving explanations relevant to social policy decisions. Moreover, the studies are done, conceptually, on series of individuals, which may make intervening at the level of individuals seem the most natural approach. It is not conceptually necessary that such studies will tend to be read as pointing in the direction of intervention at the individual level, but it is rather something like the result of a habit of thought.[3] Given that the studies were done on individuals, it may just seem that the natural way of changing someone's relationship to the world just will be to change something internal to them.

Why This Environment?

As above, if heritability estimates are to be useful, either the environment in which the estimate was generated must be assumed to be stable, or assumptions must be made about the way the genotypes in question will respond to various environments with respect to the organisms' phenotypes. Given the wide variety of phenotypes studied by human genetics researchers for which heritability estimates are generated, and the all but complete lack of relevant information about how they respond to environmental variation, the latter option seems closed off. And, as will emerge below in the discussion of various possible ways to support an assumption of environmental stability, it seems more likely that it is the assumption of environmental stability that is being made by the researchers involved.[4]

What *could be* the argument for assuming that the current environment, including contemporary culture and social systems, is not going to change much? Again, without the assumption that they will not, or assumptions about the way the genotypes in question will respond to changes in the environment, it is unclear that any study whose goal is to generate estimates of broad-sense heritability or find associations between genes and complex traits doing direct sequencing and extensive biochemical pathway analysis of the plausible pathways would be worth pursuing. After all, without such assumptions, such studies generate only very local estimates with little predictive or explanatory power. However, as the practitioners of such research don't feel the need to defend the view that the environment isn't going to change enough to make their results worthless, puzzling out from where this view of environmental stability emerges represents something of a challenge.

One possible view is that the current environment—taken to mean the current social structure of contemporary culture—is pretty much inevitable, at least in its broad outlines. This is the tack that many sociobiologists have taken, and it is one that is echoed in other accounts. Current gender inequalities and stereotypic gender roles, especially, seem susceptible to treatment as somehow "inevitable" and "natural."

Lewontin et al. quote Wilson as stating that, given our species' evolutionary history, "even in the most free and egalitarian of future societies men are likely to continue to play a disproportionate role in political life, business, and science" (Lewontin et al. 1984, 20). This sort of view has become distressingly common. Danielle Crittenden, in an editorial in the *New York Times*, claimed that women's average pay would always be lower then men's, because men and women had different "genetic wiring" that caused them to spend different amounts of time on child care and their careers. That "no women" but at least some men are "unaffected by the birth of" their child is, she claimed, "an issue to take up with nature" (Crittenden 1995) and not something we can or even should try to do anything about as a society.

Current economic systems and social inequalities in the distribution of wealth are also taken to be natural, to be "genetically hardwired" in some sense. Herrnstein and Murray's insistence that it is the high heritability of IQ and the high correlation between IQ and social success that makes social success heritable is just the latest in a long line of theories using a sort of biological determinism to support current social inequalities (see esp. Lewontin et al. 1984, chapters 1 and 4). It is, they claim, just the inevitable results of "the market economy" that "put intelligence on the sales block" and resulted in current inequalities (Herrnstein and Murray 1994, 98–99). Wilson takes the tight conceptual links between contemporary game-theoretic/economic views of adaptationist evolution and contemporary late capitalism as a starting place and claims that for the most part "members of human societies . . . compete for the limited resources" available and that this results in the "best and most entrepreneurial [gaining] a disproportionate share of rewards" (Wilson, quoted in Lewontin et al. 1984, 245).

This approach has many unlikely features. Even if it were true that in its broadest outlines (e.g., late capitalism) the current social structure was somehow inevitable, it would still not be enough to make the conclusions traditionally drawn from behavioral genetics studies follow. There is, even within the United States today, too much environmental variation available for any such conclusions to nontrivially follow. Even among monozygotic twins reared together, that one twin has some particular complex behavioral trait never guarantees that the other twin will; recall that in the behaviors and other traits the previous chapters concentrated on, the "concordance rates" (the fraction of the time the twins would share the trait) were almost always below .5, and usually much lower. This would seem to point toward the importance of the environment in the etiologies of these behaviors. If different enough environments already exist within the culture, and indeed within the same family, to influence the etiologies of the behaviors and other complex trait variations that these sorts of research projects attempt to explain, claiming that the current distributions of environments is inevitable is revealed as a strikingly bold, and indeed implausible, claim.

Further, it is worth keeping in mind that environmental changes get made all the time in our culture, and that some of these are the sort we would expect might radically alter the heritability of some traits, and indeed the relationship between genes and phenotypes. The environment of a child growing up today in a well-off American household is very different from the environment of a child growing up a few decades ago in a household of (adjusted) equal income. For example, thinking only of the ubiquity of powerful personal computers, of home entertainment centers, and the reduction in the prevalence of quality daily newspapers, one gets a very different picture of the ways that children today, in at least some households, are exposed to the world.

But no particularly good argument has ever been put forward that the current social structure and stereotypical gender roles are, even in the broadest outline, anything like "natural" or inevitable. Understood narrowly, there is no unique social structure in existence now, and insofar as there is a "Western" culture, it is a relatively recent invention, and rapidly changing. Even in terms of basic behavioral patterns, there is no evidence that the basic structure is inevitable, nor that any basic structure would be more "natural" than others. One cannot, for example, take even the ubiquity of a behavior in a given culture as evidence for it having a genetic component (see for example Lewontin 1993, 94–95).

Another approach is to claim, or to insinuate, that while perhaps not inevitable, the current situation is the best possible. This can take the form of arguing that it is the best absolutely, or, more often, that it is the best stable system when issues of fairness and justice are coupled with economic efficiency. This is the approach Jensen took in "How Much Can We Boost IQ and Scholastic Achievement?" (1969) and which Herrnstein and Murray took in *The Bell Curve* (1994). The basic line is that while things may not be perfect, and certainly are not fair in any "absolute sense" (Jensen's phrase), they are as fair, and perhaps as good, as they could be. In Herrnstein and Murray's formulation, the rise of the "cognitive elite" has been "a success for the nation as a whole" and those times in the past, when the best and brightest weren't at the top of the socioeconomic scale, were both inefficient and "frustrating" for those intelligent enough to know their talents were being wasted (1994, 511). Any attempt to make the less well-off better off today would result in everyone doing worse, or at the very least in the better-off being "dragged down" more than conditions for the less well-off are improved. At the very least, it is implied that we are currently in a condition of something like Pareto-efficiency, a situation in which any attempt to make someone better off would result in someone else doing worse.[5] Indeed, it is often insinuated that this culture has already striven too hard for an undeserved equality; note for example the recent attacks on affirmative action and welfare in the United States. Herrnstein and Murray go so far as to claim that the "complex systems" that have taken over the more free-market systems of the past have resulted in the cognitively disadvantaged being ever more put-upon, and suggest the return to a semimythical 1950s America (538–45).[6] Again, Crittenden suggests that any attempt to create situations in which men and women would share more equally both in child-rearing and career advancement is either doomed to failure, or would have associated costs that are unacceptable.

This position, though, is at best highly contentious. If the current sociocultural environment is the best one possible, if the excesses of late capitalism aren't excesses at all, then perhaps changing the environment in ways that would destroy the validity of heritability studies would be either impossible, too costly, or perhaps even unjust. But then the reason why working to change, for example, our culture's conceptions of proper gender roles or its conception of sexuality is the wrong thing to do, cannot have anything to do with the "naturalness" of the current system as revealed through heritability estimates, genes found, or sociobiological stories, on pain of circularity. If heritability estimates have meaning because of the "justness" of current practices, appealing to those same estimates to show the "justness" of current systems is obviously a grossly unacceptable move (more on this below).

Until persuasive reasons why this particular set of cultural beliefs and practices are the best possible, without recourse to sociobiological stories or studies from behavioral genetics, are forthcoming, there is no reason to accept the claim that it would be impossible, or even difficult, to make change in the broad social environment that would make current heritability estimates worthless. Rather, the conservative nature of the current heritability estimates and the use of sociobiological storytelling must be acknowledged.

Organisms as Active, Environments as Unstable

Many authors have pointed out that organisms are not the passive recipients of environmental stresses in the way that the traditional habit of thought to emerge from the modern synthesis might imply. Rather, most organisms are actively involved in choosing and modifying their environments. In examining the ways in which organisms construct and actively select their environments, both literally and metaphorically, and the ways in which environments should be thought of as unstable, this section will be pointing toward ways in which the current practices of research that claim to discover a genetic basis of variation in complex human traits are misguided, and misguided in a particularly serious and dangerous way.

The environment of an organism cannot be identified without observing its behavior in the world. That is, figuring out which parts of the world are parts of an organism's environment is not something that can be done except by observing the organism's relationship with its world (Levins and Lewontin 1985, 98–99; Brandon 1990, 68). Much of the world is irrelevant to any given organism, and figuring out which parts are relevant to it is an empirical matter, often of significant complexity. Some elements of the environment that are irrelevant for much of an organism's life can, during brief periods, become supremely relevant; consider for example nest-building behaviors or certain plants' requirements for rare environmental events in order to reproduce. Levins and Lewontin note that as the niche of an organism is a "description . . . in terms of the life activity of the [organism in question]," the concept of unoccupied niches is deeply problematic (1985, 98; see also Brandon 1990, 68). As there is an "uncountable infinity of ways" in which "the external world can be divided up," the number of possible niches is equally vast (Levins and Lewontin 1985, 68). Organisms simply do not find themselves in a preexisting niche that they must passively accept and to which natural selection works to fit the species (Levins and Lewontin 1985; Brandon 1990). Rather, organisms themselves define their niches, actively selecting from the infinite possibilities those parts of the world that, in attending to, they form their lives out of (Levins and Lewontin 1985; see Hutchinson 1965 for the classic statement of this principle).

The claim that organisms actively select their environments has at least a more figurative and more literal form. The more figurative form is hinted at above: Organisms, by living their lives in such a way that they attend to some parts of the world and ignore others, "select" from the infinite possibilities in the world a niche that they live in (Levins and Lewontin 1985, 68). This sense of "selection," though, is indeed at best figurative. More literally, however, many organisms *move*, and in doing so *literally* select the environment in which they live.[7] Odling-Smee cites Kettlewell's work on salt-and-pepper moths, noting that darker moths settle on the darker areas of trees more often than would be expected by chance (Odling-Smee 1988, 76). Prosaically, animals choose, in some loose sense of the word, the parts of the day during which they will be active. More dramatically, many mostly aquatic mammals choose how much time they spend in water versus on land, and adapt this behavior to current conditions (sea lions in California versus those in Alaska, for example). And Lewontin notes that the sea lions' "problem" of living in an aquatic environment was created by the ancestors of sea lions, and that their evolutionary development as mostly aquatic creatures was the result of their environment *becoming* increasingly aquatic, due not to changes in the world per se but rather to changes in the way they lived their lives.

But these metaphorical and literal senses of the way organisms select their environments leave out what is perhaps the most important way in which thinking of the organism as separable from its environment is problematic. It is not just that organisms choose their environments, nor even that they simply change the environments they are in as a result of, for example, consuming resources and the like. Rather, they actively create environments, physically modifying the world in ways that change their relationship to it. It is in this sense that we should think of organisms as actively constructing their environments. Odling-Smee notes that many organisms physically construct such things as "nests, burrows, paths, dams, [and] pheromone trails," and, perhaps more importantly, many organisms also "provision various 'nursery' environments for their offspring" (Odling-Smee 1988, 76, following Waddington, various). Many organisms come into a world already heavily modified for their benefit; they are given resources in ways that simply do not occur without the active participation of other organisms. Expressing this nongenetic inheritance in a model in which the environment and organism are kept strictly separate is quite tricky (see for example Odling-Smee 1988, 77).

While it is, Odling-Smee claims, "quite widely recognized" that "organisms can modify selection forces in their own environments," there is no clear consensus on what implications should be drawn from this (1988, 78). On one interpretation, though, the ability of organisms to modify their own environments in such radical ways makes the strict separability of environment from organism that is presupposed by most interpretations of the modern synthesis an unlikely, and potentially problematic, assumption. Organisms, in this view, must be thought of as integrated into their environments such that, to put it crudely, there is not even a firm border between organism and environment (see for example Odling-Smee 1988; Oyama 1985; Lewontin 1978; Levins and Lewontin 1985).

The simple view of environmental change encouraged by the modern synthesis made it out to be mostly independent of the organisms whose evolution it influenced. The working assumption of such researchers, as

Levins and Lewontin point out, is to think of environmental change in terms of "cosmological, geological, and meteorological events that have their own laws, independent of the life and death" of the organisms involved (1985, 87). Given such a view, heritability estimates might have some use, at least in human populations in advanced Western cultures, whose members are, to various degrees, shielded from such sources of change. Or, more plausibly, such changes might be thought of as long-term in scope and effect, and hence disconnected from heritability estimates, which are about what is going on *now* and for the next couple of generations at most, which after all is all that is ever considered in policy decisions.

But given even the most trivialized view of the way humans, especially, create environments for themselves and their children, such a position would be revealed as absurd. Whatever changes still occur, even mostly independently of the actions of people (and it isn't clear that any but the very fewest do),[8] the *effects* of such changes are mediated by the social systems we have created. The amount that, for example, an earthquake changes the way people live, and influences the broad organization of a society, depends vitally on where it occurs, and what had been built there. Hurricane Mitch killed over ten thousand people in 1998 primarily not because it was particularly powerful when it struck land, but rather because of *where* it struck, namely in places that couldn't be effectively evacuated and were very susceptible to damage from the massive rainfall (see McKinley and Stevens 1998). The effect that changes in weather patterns will have on a society depend on how such changes affect, for example, farming or fishing practices, and these changes are not given by the environment *simpliciter*, but from the interaction of the environment with the societies that have been formed.

But most changes in the environments that peoples are born into, grow up in, and live in are much more closely linked to people's actions in the world and less on anything resembling the autonomous changing environment often presupposed—in practice if not in principle—by evolutionary theory interpreted through the modern synthesis. Again, contra a view of our environment as basically stable, a view necessary for much of what is done in using genetics to explain differences in complex human traits that matter to us to make sense, the environment we live in is constantly changing in vast and mostly unpredictable ways. And insofar as what skills are relevant to living successful lives change as the environment changes, heritability studies and gene linkages are obviously going to be of little explanatory interest. For human behavior, especially, what makes something a skill, or even a trait worth studying or commenting upon, is the way it is wrapped up in broader social contexts. As these broader social contexts are, at least in modern Western societies, unstable, what is going to count as a skill, and what traits are going to count as worth explaining at all, will change as the environments change.

The importance of this point cannot be overstated. Lewontin's examples about the ubiquity of inexpensive calculators changing what sorts of mathematical skills are interesting and necessary and the diminishing importance of physical strength for many jobs are telling (1993, 29–30). A genetically influenced ability to do basic math quickly and accurately would no longer be worth very much, because anyone with any skill at all, when equipped with a calculator or spreadsheet program is, essentially, able to do any basic math very rapidly and with perfect accuracy—indeed, data-entry skills are now more relevant to doing basic math properly than mathematical skill per se. Changing technology and social preferences have made many previously important skills useless, and created opportunities for new skills to be created. If there are genes that influence one's ability to do high-level computer programming, they were clearly not doing *that*, and quite possibly not doing much of anything, before the advent of computers.[9]

Our ability to change our environment radically and indeed to change what traits are going to be important to us and how this importance is going to play out makes the view of organisms as separate from their environment particularly poorly suited to the analysis of human behavior. While such views may permit the mathematical modeling of changes in populations through natural selection, they are clearly of no, or at best extremely limited, use in dealing with human populations. It is not just that there are deep theoretical problems with such views in general, but that in this specific case, the assumptions they are premised on are not merely false, but absurd.

Closing the Circles

In many of the cases explored in previous chapters, a main issue was the way in which environmental changes, changes that would have the effect of bringing the validity of the research done into question, were assumed to be impossible. Ironically, the very reason such changes are assumed to be impossible is often the results of those same studies. A high heritability for a trait is assumed to reveal that most environmental changes would have no influence on that trait; that is, that the trait is either impossible to change much (as Jensen thinks of IQ), or can only be changed by directed medical intervention at the individual biochemical level (as many people think of mood-affective disorders). From this, it is supposed to follow that those broad social environments that the trait is wrapped up in are also fixed. So for example, in the case of IQ, it was the relative ranking of various kinds of groups, either "racial" or class-based, that would remain unchanged (see Murray and Herrnstein 1994, quoted above). And from this, of course, it is thought to follow that the sorts of social changes that would call the results of the studies into question are impossible. The heritability of IQ might fail in a more egalitarian society, but since power resources are always going to be distributed unequally and weighted toward those with high IQs, this form of egalitarianism will be at best very unstable, and is perhaps impossible. The circle is complete: IQ is highly heritable, so IQ can't be changed; the distribution of social positions follows from the IQ distribution, so the distribution of social positions can't be changed; since the distribution of social positions can't be changed, the high heritability of IQ in this environment can be assumed to hold in any future environments in which we might find ourselves.

The circularity is rarely that obvious, although the stories told by Herrnstein and Murray and by Jensen certainly get close. However, that kind of circularity lurks behind many uses of sociobiological storytelling, many attempts to estimate broad-sense heritability of traits in human populations, and many of the various searches for genes linked to those behavioral traits within the normal range of human behavior. No such studies, after all, could be used to help make changes. As Lewontin points out (contra Jensen), finding out how much "IQ and scholastic achievement" can be boosted is a matter of experimenting with various educational and social policies, not of searching for genes and genetic causes (Lewontin 1993, 35; see also chapter 4). Those projects involved in finding genes and even partially elucidating biochemical pathways have done little to suggest ways in which the traits in question can be changed; indeed, those projects involved in finding estimates of broad-sense heritability and sociobiological storytelling have in general set the dialogue on changing traits back. They have done this by creating the impression, generally false, that they have *shown* that the traits are somehow not amenable to environmental intervention, or could only be changed with enormous difficulty (again, see for example Hamer and Copeland 1998, 245).

Embracing Complexity

Research into the partial genetic etiologies of complex human traits should be approached with great caution and no small degree of skepticism. As it stands, for such research to be seen as explanatory requires implausible assumptions regarding environmental stability, and especially the stability of the social environment. Further, such research tends to assume that the traits being studied are somehow "natural" or "obvious" and ignores the role that our social environment plays in shaping our conception of what traits are of interest. Until research into, for example, human behavior genetics does not embrace these assumptions, they will do little more than reinforce social stereotypes and make various aspects of the status quo look natural. Other possible research programs, which take more seriously the complex interactions between the organism and its environment, including the role of the organism in modifying its own environments and the ability of organisms to respond actively to changes in their environments,[10] are much less susceptible to this sort of misuse. Whatever advantages ignoring the organism's affects on its environment and thinking in terms of "additive" genetic effects might have in terms of simplicity, when programs born out of such disregard are applied to those complex traits that matter to people living in complex societies, the results can only be unsatisfying and, ultimately, destructive.

Again, though, this is not to say that we should expect these other, more complex projects in biology to give us the kinds of answers we might want. Finding out how to explain the source of those human variations that are important to us, and how to predict what kinds of changes will influence these differences, may well be beyond the current "state of the art" in human genetics research. But of course, we should not be satisfied with simplistic environmental or cultural explanations either. Rather, we ought to recognize that explaining these sorts of differences, and predicting these kinds of effects, is probably well beyond any simple method.

Does this mean that we ought to give up, that we ought to despair? I think not. If we cannot, for reasons of intellectual honesty, permit ourselves to be guided by either the findings of simplistic and conceptually flawed research into the relationship between human genetics and complex traits, or by equally simplistic and misguided "environmental" explanations of these important variations, we are still not forbidden from making changes, from trying different things and seeing what works, from trying out different kinds of complex explanations, and seeing which ones we can use to best make sense of our lives. Someday, perhaps, science will be able to give us firm answers to those questions about human variations that we really want answered; perhaps eventually science will answer such questions as, How *do* we make our children as smart as they can be, as healthy as they can be, physically and mentally? How *do* we make our cities safer without needlessly infringing on important liberties? (And so on.) Right now, I think, science cannot do that, and we would be much better off turning to other sources of inspiration than pretending that it can.

NOTES

Chapter 1

1. The headlines were all taken from the *New York Times*. They were: Associated Press 1997, "Gene Discovery May Yield Test for Glaucoma"; Grady, D. 1997a, "Brain-Tied Gene Defect May Explain Why Schizophrenics Hear Voices"; Grady, D. 1997b, "Finding Genetic Traces of Jewish Priesthood"; Angier, N. 1996a, "People Haunted by Anxiety Appear to Be Short on a Gene"; Leary, W. E. 1996, "Scientists Identify Site of Gene Tied to Some Cases of Parkinson's"; *New York Times* 1996, "Gene May Be Clue to Nature of Nurturing"; Blakeslee, S. 1996, "Researchers Track Down a Gene That May Govern Spatial Abilities"; Kolata, G. 1996, "Is a Gene Making You Read This?"; Angier, N. 1996b, "Variant Gene Tied to a Love of New Thrills."

2. Except perhaps for physical abnormalities and diseases, most of the complex traits of interest in human genetic research are behavioral. And, further, it seems unlikely that the level of interest and excitement about human genetic research would be as great if it were only physical abnormalities and diseases that were at issue.

Chapter 2

1. Bailey lists this, the "fallacy of useless intervention," as one of the five major fallacies of "hereditarian science" (see Bailey 1997, 126). This is closely related to what Kitcher refers to as "the crudest sort of genetic determinism"—the claim that "norm of reaction for the trait of interest is flat" (1999, 5). This articulation of genetic determinism will be become clearer in the next chapter, where the concept of a "norm of reaction" is introduced.

2. Kitcher points out that what I am calling the "methodological" thesis can be entirely disassociated from the causal thesis (1998, 23). This point was also made clear to me by Stephen Downes.

3. This is a common interpretation. See for example also Cantor 1992, Hood 1992, and Caskey 1992.

4. It is this sort of claim which makes it clear that it is the above-mentioned "intervention is useless" strand of genetic determinism that is being argued against by reference to PKU.

5. In Plomin et al. 1997 they tell much the same story:
   PKU was found to be a single-gene cause of mental retardation. . . . An environmental intervention was successful in bypassing the genetic problem of high levels of

phenylalanine: Administer a diet low in phenylalanine. This important environmental intervention was made possible by recognition of the genetic basis for this type of mental retardation. (85)

PKU is the best example of the usefulness of finding genes for behavior. Knowledge that PKU is caused by a single gene led to an understanding of how the genetic defect causes mental retardation. (111)

6. One could be forgiven for thinking that many of these authors know very little about PKU, and are simply repeating some version of the myth they've read or been told. To claim, as for example Nelkin and Dawkins do, that the dietary measures are "rather simple" and "easy" reveals either a complete lack of knowledge about what is involved in feeding children a low-phenylalanine diet or a rather different concept of "simple" and "easy" than most of us have. Low-phenylalanine diets are exceedingly unpleasant, have problematic relationships to other key nutrients, and are correlated with emotional problems and behavioral disorders in the children receiving them (see Scriver et al. 1988, 311ff.; Paul 1994 makes a similar point). The suggestion in Greely's telling of the tale that it is the affected persons themselves who modify their diets seems to be simply a bizarre slip.

7. Murphey writes that "although a simplistic concept of PKU genetics was heuristically useful in the past, the belief may now have outlived its value" (1982, 141). Fifteen years later, Vigue still writes of PKU as if it were that sort of "winsome example of fact" (see above). If, as I claim below, the usefulness of the simplistic PKU story comes not primarily from its being a heuristically useful set of beliefs to guide research, but rather as part of the storytelling tradition of behavioral genetics itself, its value obviously remains as great now as ever.

8. Perhaps even more interesting, in Plomin et al. 1997 the more detailed story is excluded. Instead, the story told about PKU is a "hybrid" between what Murphey calls the "myth" and more precise formulations.

9. Fölling's "The Discovery of Phenylketonuria" (1994) provides an interesting variation on the standard story. In this version (told by the son of Asbjörn Fölling, the discoverer of PKU), there is a much heavier concentration on the details of the chemistry than is usually given.

10. The effectiveness of the low-phenylalanine diets was thrown into some doubt by the existence of individuals with high-phenylalanine blood levels but normal mentation (especially since the mean IQ of those on a low-phenylalanine diet is still somewhat below average). Studies of siblings in which the older siblings were not treated (because the treatments hadn't been developed yet) while the younger children were treated pointed convincingly toward the diet's effectiveness (the studies suggest that the diet is at least partially effective in preventing retardation, especially in radically reducing the number of individuals with severe mental retardation) (Plomin 1990, 82–83). More recent studies and developments in the treatment of PKU (the careful monitoring of the relationship between tyrosine and phenylalanine levels, increased treatment lengths, etc.) have steadily brought the IQ and number of other developmental problems associated with PKU closer to the population average. It has become clear that proper management of PKU is not just a matter of "simple" diet modification, but of careful monitoring and biochemical adjustments, often throughout the life of the individual (see the American Academy of Pediatrics Committee on Genetics, "Newborn Screening Fact Sheet, 1996.)

There is some doubt about what percentage of individuals with blood-serum phenylalanine levels in the "classic PKU" range or mutations associated with a complete or nearly complete inability to metabolize phenylalanine will have, for example, normal mental functioning. More on this below.

11. On this topic see for example, Lewontin 1993, esp. 67ff.

Below, I argue that the claim is made that medical treatments grow out of understanding the genetics of conditions more often than is actually the case. However, it is important to keep in mind that *some* medical treatments really do emerge from understanding the genetics (many of the treatments developed in AIDs research, for example, grew out of an attention to the molecular level).

12. Paul (1994) makes a similar point, claiming that PKU was *not* a success for genetic medicine, but rather only for genetic testing.

13. Indeed, a quick Medline search reveals an enormous and growing number of articles listing new defects in the PAH (phenylalanine hydroxylase) and BH(4) coding regions correlated with PKU and other forms of hyperphenylalaninemia. Scriver's "Whatever Happened to PKU?" (1995) gives a good summary of some of the more important results up to mid-1990s.

14. Cystic fibrosis is also genetically and clinically heterogeneous. This explains, in part, why estimates of how much it cost to "find the CF gene" vary so much. Some take the first form found (which is present in some 70-plus percent of chromosomes carrying the CF mutation) as finishing the task; others consider the search still on. See James Watson citing Francis Collins as claiming a $10–50 million cost (1992, 169). Hood estimates the cost of the search as closer to $150 million (1992, 158) and, oddly enough, in 1989 Francis Collins told the Senate that the search for the CF gene cost well over $400 million (though it is difficult to assess just what he was counting as money spent aiding the search); (Collins 1989, 69).

15. Attempts have been made to find ways to tie the treatment into the genetic discoveries, but these have been unconvincing at best. See Ledley 1991 for a discussion. See for example Treacy et al. 1996, Rasmus et al. 1993, and Tyfield et al. 1990 for some case studies that reveal the difficulties with such a plan.

It is interesting that the faith that information about genes influences treatments crops up in so many different places where there is no reason to believe it is the case. Wilson, in the above-quoted letter to *Nature*, claims that racism could be circumvented by knowledge of its hereditary basis "*just as* a knowledge of the hereditary basis of haemoglobin chemistry and insulin production can lead to the amelioration of the pathological variants" (1981, 627, emphasis added). But, again, the treatments for insulin-dependent diabetes, for example, were developed well before the genetics of the disease were understood, and had nothing to do with an attention to them.

16. Paul 1994 cites Acuff and Faden 1991 for the 90 percent figure. Acuff and Faden actually give the figure as 95 percent, and fail to give any reference for it at all. The failure is striking in part because every other claim made in the paragraph in which the number is given is referenced. It is likely that Acuff and Faden got the number from the "Newborn Screening Fact Sheet" (1989, 1996), which they cite several times, and which also gives the number as 95 percent. The "Newborn Screening Fact Sheet" gives no reference for that number, however.

Chapter 3

1. I am uncomfortable with this way of describing "heritability," for reasons that will become clear below; it is, however, the standard description (see for example Crow 1986; Plomin et al. 1990). As should be clear, the word "attributable" is a big part of the difficulty; it isn't at all clear that any good sense can be made of this. However, other formulations that lack this problem are very awkward.

Broad-sense heritability, H^2, is distinguished from *narrow-sense* heritability, h^2. Narrow-sense heritability is the phenotypic variance "attributable" (in the sense described below) to the effects of *additive* genetic loci *only* (e.g., it excludes those involved in such phenomena as dominance, epistasis, and genetic covariances). It is of some interest in plant and animal breeding, but is of little interest for explaining or making predictions about human variation. Many of the objections to inappropriate uses of broad-sense heritability below apply equally well to uses of narrow-sense heritability; however, it is somewhat rarer that narrow-sense heritability is misinterpreted in the ways described below.

2. This discussion follows Lewontin (1974), Plomin et al. (1990), and Crow (1986). The term "e," the "everything else" term, is often taken to be a combination of developmental noise (the effect of irreducible randomness on the developmental process) and unique environmental experiences (differences in the environmental experiences of, say, lab animals where the environments have been made as similar as is possible; those environmental variations that cannot be quantified). This term, "e," is often deliberately excluded (see Kitcher 1999 for an argument that those variations ought to be, at best, thought of as artifacts of our lack of knowledge). GE is often excluded for convenience (see Plomin et al. 1990, 227), though I will argue below that excluding GE cannot, in general, be defended.

   This equation assumes the independence of the variables. This means that (for example) organisms with a certain genotype are no more likely than any others to be in any particular environment, or vice versa. Examples where independence fail are common in nature (see for example Odling-Smee 1988, Lewontin 1978). More on this below.

3. Kitcher refers to this as an "unfortunate tic" from which the behavioral genetics community is unable to free itself (Kitcher 1999, 22, n. 11).

4. Crow notes that Wright developed "a scale transformation that makes the variance [in white spotting] independent of the amount of white" (Crow 1986, 126); hence, what the actual units refer to is somewhat obscure in this example. It is, however, of no importance to the point of the example.

5. This example was developed in large part in an exchange with Peter Godfrey-Smith in 1995–96. The discussion of this experiment that takes place in chapter 4 also owes much to that exchange.

   I assume throughout that "e" (developmental noise, unique environmental experience, and error) is equal to 0.

6. A slight complication is that the maze-bright and maze-dull rats that Cooper and Zubek did not form two genetically homogeneous groups—each group probably represented a diverse population, genetically speaking. Rather than thinking of each population as representing a particular *genotype*, though, one might think of the two groups of rats as representing distinct *ecotypes*, populations specifically adapted to particular environmental circumstances. Due to the selective pressures, the maze-bright rats were adapted to an environment in which running mazes well resulted in reproductive success, and, oddly enough, the maze-dull rats were specifically "adapted" to an environment in which running mazes poorly yielded reproductive success.

7. Plomin et al. do not present this example in their 1997 edition.

8. But see above on problems with the population interpretation taken to be informative about what would happen in populations with reduced genetic and/or environmental variation. However, in this case, since we are speaking of large numbers of genetically heterogenous men and an environmental distribution that is a subset of the previous one, this problem is perhaps not so pressing. This is especially true of Crow, who has, in the section in which this example occurs, abstracted away from considerations of genotype-environment covariances and other complications (Crow 1986, 124).

9. As Crow is explicitly abstracting away from the possible covariance of genotypes and environments here, he cannot, even in principle, assume the above kind of covariance.

10. In this case, both heritability and environmentality are equal to about .19.

11. Once again, the actual numbers used are squared to generate *variances*, for technical reasons, and this shared difference is referred to as the amount that the organisms *covary*. In this case,

heritability is simply the amount of *covariation* in the population divided by the total pheno-typic variation.

12. Most experiments of this type actually use genetically identical animals or plants generated through selective crossbreeding programs rather than through cloning, because of the technical difficulties with reliably cloning most experimental animals; even many plants are difficult to reliably clone in vitro.

13. Bailey (1997) develops several compelling (and quite interesting) examples in which measured heritability will be misleading in the extreme.

14. This discussion follows Lewontin 1974 very closely. Griffiths et al. 1996 provide additional illuminating examples based on the same basic ideas.

15. *Allometry* relates the size (or other measure) of some organ or feature to changes in the size (or other measure) of some other organ or feature (including, for example, overall size). Allometric changes are thought to be responsible for much of the complex integration of organisms. See Schlichting and Pigliucci 1998, 85–109.

16. This is of course merely a vastly simplified sketch meant to give a rough idea of what "finding a gene" entails. Readers interested in the fascinating details of these processes may wish to start with Judson's "A History of the Science and Technology behind Gene Mapping and Sequencing" (1992), a very readable introduction to the subject. Readers wishing more detail may wish to consider *An Introduction to Genetic Analysis*, (Griffiths et al. 1996), an excellent basic text that also contains a quite perspicuous discussion of heritability and reactions norms.

17. Some relatively recent discoveries include genes associated with Huntington's disease, Alzheimer's disease, and early-onset breast cancer. There are thousands of diseases with a known genetic component (around five thousand is a common estimate of the number of known genetic diseases—see Caskey 1992 and Wexler 1992), and in many cases the genes associated with them have been found and sequenced.

18. What constitutes part of the spectrum of the "normal" and what constitutes an "abnormal" condition is actually a hard problem, but not one we need be terribly concerned with here (see chapter 6, "Gay Genes and the Reification of Homosexuality," for some comments on how this problem plays out in a specific case). Readers interested in following up on this topic may find Canguilhem's *The Normal and the Pathological* (1991) and the collection edited by Caplan et al., *Concepts of Health and Disease* (1981), of interest. In any event, the simple heritable diseases discussed above are pretty uncontroversial.

19. In this use of the term, epistatic effects are to be thought of as *physiological;* in an individual organism, there is, at the biochemical level, a mechanistic interaction between the gene products that influences the traits in question. This is as opposed to, for example, Fisher's use of the term, where it is a "statistical phenomenon" with "no necessary reflection at the gene level" (Schlichting and Pigliucci 1998, 6–7).

20. See Chorney et al. 1998 and various press reports of the discovery of "a locus associated with cognitive ability," or as the *New York Times* would have it, "a gene associated with high intelligence" (Wade 1998). This research is discussed in more detail in the next chapter.

21. See for example Lewontin et al. 1984; Lewontin 1993; Kitcher 1985; Fausto-Sterling 1985; and Dupré 1997. Many of the criticisms of sociobiological accounts of human behaviors stem from (a) the lack of empirical data for the universal existence traits proposed, and especially the lack of good, consistent cross-cultural and cross-temporal data; (b) the apparent ease of telling stories that can account for any and all behaviors encountered; (c) the variety of other possible explanations that can account for the same data; (d) the lack of any evidence that there was genetically induced variation in the traits at some point for there to

have been selection on; and, more generally (e) the lack of evidence for any plausible developmental pathway from the hypothesized genes to the trait.

22. Exceptions to this general rule are sociobiological accounts of the differences between the sexes in humans (see Buss 1994, etc.), where arguments about different mating strategies being pursued by the males and females are commonplace, and arguments about different abilities (or levels of ability) in males and females having a biological basis that emerges out of the genetics (see Dupré 1997, Longino 1990, Fausto-Sterling 1985 for critiques of these programs).

23. While from the standpoint of certain mathematical approaches to modeling evolution these two sources of variation (individuals who can vary their response versus mixed populations of individuals who always play the same strategy) can often be treated as interchangeable (see for example Skyrms 1996 and references therein), it should be obvious that they are *not* equivalent from a causal point of view. In one case, the variation that exists is supposed to be the result of genetic variation *between* individuals; in the other case, it is supposed that the variation could result from the genetically controlled plasticity of a single genotype to the different (e.g., developmental) environments encountered.

24. Readers interested in the way that these sorts of arguments can be formalized and the computer simulations of the systems run may find Skyrms 1996 and the references therein of interest. One lesson that can be learned from reading Skyrms is that how these hypothetical systems are formalized is (a) pretty much up for grabs and (b) matters to the results. In this case, it would be a relatively easy task to find some mathematicalization of the hypothesized situation that would yield the desired results.

25. Hamer and Copeland write, "This . . . may well explain why there is still such great variation in the D4DR gene in modern day humans" (1998, 49). I think we ought to be inclined to argue that while we have no evidence that the variation in the D4DR gene is *not* the result of an evolutionarily stable polymorphism, we also have no evidence that it *is* the result of one, which should I think dampen our enthusiasm for such phrases as "may well explain" and the like.

    This move, from "it is possible that x," to "therefore, x may well explain y" or "perhaps x explains y" is made often in the literature on using evolutionary reasoning to account for complex human traits (see for example Skryms 1996). Where it is unclear (as it is here) that the thing to be explained stands in need of the sort of explanation offered, and it is unclear that any evidence for the truth of the explanation could be gathered, the point of these arguments (beyond the rhetorical) is often hard to see.

Chapter 4

1. I will continue to use the rather cumbersome locution "performance on IQ tests" rather than speaking of IQs *simpliciter* because, while I do not deal with the problem here, the question of what IQ tests actually measure and what the scores that are generated on them refer to (if anything) strikes me as remaining something of an open one.

2. Sober notes that a trait may perform some useful task even where the performance of that task is not implicated in the evolution of the trait in question (1993, 84). A trait may do something, say, *t*, as a "spinoff" of its evolutionarily explanatory "use" and there would have been *selection of t*'ers but no *selection for t*-ing, to use Sober's terminology (1993, 83). In this case, one might wish to consider what traits were being *selected for* (low error rates) in Sober's sense, and what had merely experienced a "spinoff" *selection-of.*

3. I will continue to refer to "races" in scare-quotes, despite serious misgivings about using the notion at all in this context. Modern population genetics of the sort most often associated with Cavalli-Sforza seem to point toward the concept of "race" being of at best very

ambiguous value in thinking about genetic differentiation among human populations. The complexities in this attack on the concept of "race" are, however, extreme, since in populations such as the United States, where much of the continuum between those variations in distributions of genotypic traits between, for example, people of northern European descent and people of African descent is missing (not because it doesn't exist at all, but because peoples with those sorts of distributions don't yet make up a sizable percentage of the current population of the United States), "race" is an occasionally useful category for thinking about, for example, risk factors for certain genetic diseases. That this should not be taken to imply that there is anything metaphysically "deep" about the notion of "race" should be obvious, but getting clear on exactly what sorts of uses of "race" are valuable (e.g., some sociological and some epidemiological uses) and what sort are actively pernicious (e.g., arguments about genetic inferiority) would take us rather far afield.

4. In however strong or trivial a sense of "because of genetic differences" one likes. Consider a culture (like Apartheid-era South Africa) in which "racial" facts, however socially constructed, correspond however loosely to some differences in genetic distributions within the given population. In such a culture, given the radically different treatment of the identified "races," differences in genetic distributions will end up driving, in some loose sense, all kinds of differences (income, respect, likelihood of incarceration, etc.). And, this happens in a way that might be described as "because of genetic differences." Similarly, lab rats that had their legs surgically removed if they happened to have some genetic marker would have differences in their abilities to move that could be described, in some sense, as being "because of genetic differences." Whether we wish to count such indirect effects as "genetic" is, however, something of an open question, and pursuing it here would take us too far afield. (See for example Block 1995, 104; Hamer and Copeland 1998, 42–43; Dawkins 1982, 12ff.).

5. The way they arrive at this number appears only in the endnotes and is as follows: "The standard deviation of IQ being 15, the variance is therefore 225. We are stipulating that environment accounts for .4 of the variance, which equals 90. The standard deviation of the distribution of the environmental component of IQ is the square root of 90, or 9.49. The difference between group environments necessary to produce a fifteen-point difference in group means is 15/9.49, or 1.58." (Murray and Herrnstein, 724). Given their initial claim of 1.2 standard deviations, or 17 IQ points, the difference between group environments would be 1.79 standard deviations.

6. A 17-point IQ gap lowers the required percentile of the average environmental distribution of black Americans to around the 4th percentile of the average environmental distribution for white Americans. Again, it is wise to keep in mind that these numbers emerge from an attention to the area under normal (gaussian) distribution curves, and nothing more. The assumption that a normal distribution curve is the right way to model environmental distributions in the United States is, to say the least, contentious. More on this point below.

7. For example and put bluntly, even very poor white Americans are never called "nigger." Nor are they associated with the *same* stereotypes—though they are, of course, associated with different negative stereotypes. (See Omi and Winant 1986.) More locally, poor white Americans taking, for example, an intelligence test are not under the same kind of pressures from the threat of fulfilling stereotypes; see below on the power of stereotyping brought out in these sorts of situations by, for example, Steele and Aronson 1995; Steele 1997, 1998.

8. Indeed, Murray and Herrnstein have become somewhat famous for doing that in *The Bell Curve*. Most famously, perhaps, they tell, in a box on page 310, "The German Story," where they note that among the illegitimate children fathered in Germany during the Allied occupation in World War II, there was no discernible difference between the average IQ scores of the children based on the "race" of their fathers. They note that this is "consistent with the suggestion that the B/W difference is largely environmental" and then proceed to draw

the conclusion that the difference in average IQ scores of black and white Americans is unlikely to be primarily environmental, conveniently forgetting their own stories.

9. One standard deviation of IQ scores is fixed at 15 points. The difference in average IQ scores between the Dutch in 1952 and the Dutch in 1982 is 21 points. Following Murray and Herrnstein's calculations, we note that the standard deviation of IQ being 15, the variance is therefore 225. Again, if we assume that environment accounts for .4 of the variance, the variance due to the environment is once again 90. The standard deviation of the distribution of the environmental component of IQ is the square root of 90, or 9.49; 21/9.94 is about 2.21, and a quick glance at any table of normal distribution functions reveals that this corresponds to something like .9865 of the area under the curve.

   Of course, as little reason as we have to assume a heritability of performance on IQ tests of .6 in America today, we have that much less to assume any such number for the Dutch of 1952. But, again, given that almost none of the attempts to estimate the heritability of IQ in human populations have used racially mixed populations, I can see no better reason to assume any such number for black Americans than for the Dutch of 1952. Since Murray and Herrnstein permit themselves to assume that a heritability estimate that holds for white Americans will also hold for black Americans, I see no reason why in following their reasoning I shouldn't take similar liberties.

10. To be perfectly fair, Koshland's comment *may* simply have been a statement of general pessimism. But even if such pessimism is justified, it is not justified *because* of any findings in genetics.

11. A critic of Murray's who claims to share many of his libertarian views takes him to task for using a similar line of reasoning as follows: "Why . . . predict that we are not liable to change intelligence much, citing the failure of Head Start programs as proof? If government uplift debacles implied that real people could not achieve real results, then the very real failure of federal housing programs would prove the theoretical inability of modern societies to find shelter" (Hazlett 1995, 66). Bashing the government on the one hand and claiming that its failure to do something proves it can't be done on the other *does* seem a bit inconsistent.

12. I do not mean here to imply that any good sense can be made of the phrases "saner by the same amount" or even by "boosting everyone's ability to do mathematical problems by the same amount." In fact, I rather doubt that any good sense can be made of these phrases. But the point of my argument is that *even if* we accept the assumption of additivity, and the absurd consequences that seem to follow from it, the arguments about social policy that are supposed to follow still fail to.

13. It should be noted again that, quite interestingly, Murray and Herrnstein here ignore the data available on interracial adoptions (where the gap in the performance on IQ tests between white and black Americans vanishes), and the improved scores of adopted children compared to children who remain in relatively poor homes that adoption studies generally show.

14. I wish to stress here that the "if" should be taken very seriously indeed; we have no or very little evidence about the genetic variations between "races," except that there is far less genetic variation between populations than within populations (see for example Cavalli-Sforza and Cavalli-Sforza 1995 and Lewontin 1982). This data is often interpreted as implying that differences of the sort suggested by Murray and Herrnstein are implausible; however, I think it is more accurate to admit that at present there is not enough information about the relationship between genetic variation and variation in for example performance on IQ tests for us to even know where to look to find support or lack thereof for such hypotheses.

15. An interesting claim that has been made in favor of continued investigation into the genetic basis of human intellectual differences is that in the future, "teachers could be designing classes for individual children based on their genetic makeup" to maximize each student's ability to learn (Martin, quoted by Aldhous 1992, 164), basically on the hypothesis that chil-

dren's learning responses will be varied. However, given that we have no idea how we might be able to generate reaction norms for any human traits at all, let alone complex traits like "learning ability," it is unclear how this promise could be realized.

16. In fact, what we *really* want is the multifactorial reaction norm that plots all the genes involved and their interactions against all the environments involved, and *their* interactions. Whether such a thing is even conceptually possible (and it might not be—environments might not be so discretely recognizable; see chapter 10 and for example Lewontin 1978) it is certainly beyond the current capabilities of biological research (even those studies involving simple plants are rarely able to deal with more than a few factors).

Chapter 5

1. MAOA (monoamine oxidase A) is a compound that metabolizes serotonin, dopamine, and noradrenaline (all involved in neural signal transmission). In MAOA deficiency, individuals are unable to metabolize these compounds normally. The result is a variety of physical and mental disorders. More on this below. See Mann 1994; Brunner et al. 1993.

2. Ultimately, perhaps, by getting rid of the criminal genes that caused it. On this topic, see Gould on Ferri's recommendations for the "elimination" of antisocial individuals (Gould 1981, 140).

3. The use of the gender-specific "him" is deliberate, since in the advanced Western societies in question it is predominately males who are the small percentage of the population who commit the majority of the crimes (see Moffitt and Mednick 1988, preface).

4. This discounts Ferri's entirely unsupported (and somewhat bizarre) claim in 1911 that the Italian army's prescreening of recruits eliminated the practice of *misdeismo* (the "fragging" of officers—where "fragging" is a very specific way of killing an officer, usually rolling an antipersonnel grenade into his tent) during the First World War. See Gould 1981 136.

5. For some subtle biological stories, see, from Moffitt and Mednick 1988, "EEG Topography in Patients with Aggressive Violent Behavior" (V. Milstein); "Hemisphere Function in Violent Offenders" (I. Nachshon); "Psychopathy and Language" (R. D. Hare et al.); "Antisocial Behavior of Boys and Autonomic Activity/Reactivity" (D. Magnusson). For a summary of some of the even vaguer links (including MBD and abnormally low serum cholesterol), see, from the same compilation, "Biology, Mental Disorder, Aggression and Violence: What Do We Know?" (S. Hodgins and M. V. Von Grunau). DiLalla and I. Gottesman 1991 gives brief summaries of recent biological causal hypothesis (including MPAs). For critiques of such vague criteria, see for example Lewontin et al. 1984, esp. 165ff.; and Szasz 1987.

6. The extraordinary inequalities and socially enforced apartheid rioters were reacting against could just as easily be viewed as having required a more, not less, extreme response from "reasonable" people. On one view of what emerged from those times, on just how short-lasting the gains made were and the viciousness of the "conservative" response in the 1990s, the problem with the riots in the 1960s was not that *some* people engaged in violent protest, but rather that most didn't (see Omi and Winant 1994). Less controversially, there is again room to argue about whether apartheid in South Africa would have ended as quickly as it did without the activities of the African National Congress.

7. I mention this because it is often thought that politically motivated violence, in the forms of wars or organized genocides, is, because of its relative impersonality and "cleanness," somehow different from the sort of violence that makes some cities in the United States particularly unsafe. Certainly, the violence of strategic bombing is very different from the violence of a murder committed during a carjacking. However, it should be kept in mind that in much of the world political violence is still brutally personal.

Chapter 6

1. Examples of physical diseases with genetic etiologies include PKU, Huntington's disease, and cystic fibrosis. Chapter 8 argues that obesity is too often conceived of as a physical disease with a genetic etiology like these, but in any event, studies of obesity definitely aim at control of the condition, whether or not it is a "genetic disease" *simpliciter*. Similar, studies into the etiology of mental disorders like depression (see chapter 7) or schizophrenia clearly have control as their aim. The real goals of studies into antisocial behaviors such as heavily recidivist criminality and violence may be, as the last chapter argued, a bit more complex, but the stated goal is still control of the individual behavior.

2. Although Murphy, at least, seems to argue that should it become possible to predict the future sexual orientation of people prenatally, abortions of fetuses with orientations "undesired" by their parents would not be obviously morally wrong nor stand in need of legal or social prohibitions (Murphy 1997).

3. Although Bem notes that some survey data seem to imply that belief that homosexuality is biologically caused is correlated with tolerance (Bem 1996, citing Ernulf et al. 1989 and Moore 1993). However, the contrast in these surveys was primarily with homosexuality's being something like a "choice" (which is an ill-chosen contrast, as many non–biologically determined features are yet not choices). Further, Bem notes that the direction of the causal arrow remains unclear in these surveys; that is, it is unclear that tolerant people believe homosexuality not to be a choice, or that people who don't believe homosexuality to be a choice are tolerant. In any event, as I note below; the evidence that homosexuality is, in the United States (and many other Western societies; for example the United Kingdom), nothing like a "choice" and not something that can be changed by deliberate interventions is overwhelming, and the sort of toleration that would follow from homosexuality's not being a choice is the wrong sort in any event.

4. See for example Hamer and Copeland on the "consistent failure of attempts to change gay men to straight" (Hamer and Copeland 1994, 65, 109–10). Also note Halperin here on the dangers of homosexual "determinism" (either biological or psychological). Halperin reminds us that the move from treating homosexuality as a moral failing or acquired perversity to a "natural condition" in the nineteenth century resulted in the move from fixed jail terms (and the ordinary rule of law) to indefinite sentences in insane asylums (and radical medical experimentation). As long as the dominant discourse treats homosexuality as outside the normal continuum of behavior, any interpretation can be, in Halperin's terms, reconfigured to fit the dominant interests; "no account," he notes, "is so positive as to be proof against hostile appropriation and transformation" (see Halperin 1990, 52). It is at least partially for this reason that the hope that showing that sexuality is somehow innate will somehow increase social tolerance is dangerously naive.

5. Murphy, however, claims that if a "treatment for adult homoeroticism" were developed and people chose not to use it, "the reality of gay people might be driven home all the more powerfully" (1997, 58). Perhaps, but the very notion that this hypothetical thing would be properly called a "treatment" is terribly disturbing, and, to those people who believe that homosexuality is a "sickness," such a treatment, and people's refusal to use it, could, it seems, be badly misused politically (see note 3, above). Would, to foreshadow an example developed below, something that caused people who preferred chocolate to vanilla to reverse those preferences be properly described as a "treatment"? I think not.

6. On the other hand, Hamer at least claims to express an equal interest in genetic correlates to "tongue curling" ability. Any difference in interest, he seems to think, between "tongue curling" and sexual orientation comes not from their ties to other intrinsic characteristics, but to the way the latter may have implications for various health-related issues related to various sexually transmitted diseases (Hamer, personal communication). This, however,

merely highlights the differences between the opinions held by the researchers themselves and the sorts of opinions that the funding and public consumption of their results are fueled by. And again, however often Hamer insists that homosexuality is part of the normal variation in human sexual behavior, the interpretation given his results often remains independent of his own views on the issues. It should also be noted that the next molecular searches Hamer became involved in were for genes associated with "anxiety" and "novelty seeking," *not* tongue curling. While both "anxiety" and "novelty seeking" *are* what we might call constitutive features of a person's personality, "novelty seeking," at least, seems to have no medical issues directly associated with it (see Hamer and Copeland 1998, 48ff.). Perhaps, as is so often the case, Hamer is not entirely clear about his own reasons for wanting to pursue certain research topics rather than others.

7. Although larger pedigree analysis (e.g., a multigenerational family tree, with the phenotype of interest; that is, homo- or heterosexuality, noted in each case where it was known) was used in the original research and it was this larger analysis which first suggested sex linkage. See Hamer et al. 1993.

   In this context, it is interesting to note that Hamer himself recognizes that in general using sib-pair shared-trait analysis on siblings from large multigeneration pedigrees preselected for showing clear inheritance patterns, which his own research did, has the effect of skewing the correlations found toward rare, high-penetrance genes, and away from what are generally expected to be the sort of much more common low-penetrance genes implicated in most behavioral traits that have a genetic component (Hamer, personal communication). How to interpret his own research in light of this observation remains somewhat unclear; however, Hamer argues that this may in part explain the failure of Rice et al. to find linkage in the Canadian families they studied, since the research methods of Rice's team would not result in such a skewing (Hamer, quoted in Wickelgren 1999, 571; see also Rice et al. 1999).

8. Besides permitting the use of smaller family pedigrees and sample sizes, this method has the added benefit that individual mistakes are less likely to matter than in linkage studies that make use of relationships between generations. Work by Hodge and Greenberg on intergenerational linkage studies, for example, point toward the existence of "key individuals," those for whom changes in either phenotypic or genotypic assignment can radically change the resulting logarithm of odds (LOD) score. The logarithm of odds score is a measurement of the chance that the apparent linkage between a trait and a region of the genome is the result of random chance rather than a real association. It is, as the name suggests, the log (in base ten) of the odds that the association is a chance event. So, an LOD score of 3 represents a 1:1000 chance (.1 percent) that the association is not real, a LOD score of 4 represents a 1:10000 chance (.01 percent), etc. The misidentification of key individuals is apparently what happened in the Old Amish studies of manic depression, and probably accounts for many of the most disturbing cases of vanishing LOD scores. However with sib-pair methods, no individual can effect the resulting LOD score in such a radical way. See Marshall 1993.

   However, this should not be taken to mean that the sib-pair shared-trait method is without difficulties. I radically simplify Hamer's work here, ignoring such issues as his work eliminating the possibilities of such effects as segregation distortion, sexual imprinting, etc., with the sections of the chromosome in question. See Hamer and Copeland 1994. Many of the attacks on Hamer's methodology emerged from a mistrust that Hamer had in fact eliminated these possibilities in the samples he studied (Hamer did not, for example, test sibling pairs discordant for sexual orientation in the work for his first paper; see however Hu et al. 1995, where some of these early perceived shortcomings were dealt with) (see Risch et al. 1993).

9. The LOD scores for the association Hamer found were in the high 3 to low 4 range. See note 8, above, for discussion.

10. Hamer and Copeland are somewhat less modest about the research, and the chances of finding, sequencing, and interpreting "the gene" in their *Living With Our Genes* (1998).

11. Of course, actually finding out *anything* about the pathway would require finding and sequencing the gene and figuring out what the gene-product actually *did* at a biochemical/developmental level, something that hasn't yet been done for a gene associated with any complex human trait (see chapter 3).

12. It would be interesting, but not terribly relevant to the topic at hand, to explore the different sorts of sexual relationships women, slaves, and foreigners could have with each other in ancient Greek tradition. Halperin suggests that for women to place themselves in the insertive role was considered problematic, but it is unclear whether this is because of the nature of their relationships with each other (ie., that they gender themselves as male with respect to some females), or by analogy to the political problems men face when permitting themselves to be gendered as female (see Halperin 1990, 22–23). Butler's "The Lesbian Phallus and the Morphological Imaginary" (1993) is suggestive in this context. See esp. 85ff.

13. Interestingly, Whitam and Mathy imply that this concentration on the active/passive role, as opposed to the (biological) sex of the participants, is mirrored somewhat in Latin-American sexual traditions. They note that in (at least contemporary) "American homosexuals" the "activo-pasivo" distinction is "regarded as private and unimportant," whereas the first question asked of homosexual Guatemalan relationships is "Who gave ass?" However, it is not clear from Whitam and Mathy's account what role this interest plays in their relationships. See Whitam and Mathy 1986, 135.

14. I use this term in the way the term "living languages" is used; that is, to describe a system that is still vital and used, and hence open to change and in fact constantly changing, as opposed, say, to historical cultures and dead languages that (perhaps) can be thought of as rigidly definable, and certainly as "unchanging" in some sense.

15. It is sometimes suggested that the best answer to questions like Halperin's, above, is something like, "More like a gay woman who isn't into S/M in some ways, more like a straight woman who is in others" (Godfrey-Smith, for example, has suggested such an answer; personal communication, 1996). Fair enough, but as will become clearer below, the force of Halperin's question is about the immediate ways in which we see and categorize other people and ourselves, and the extent to which these categories influence other aspects of our lives. In this culture, being gay is clearly the more "basic" category of analysis, and, as Fadermen notes, often carries with it "an entire social life" (Faderman 1994, 17) in a way that being into S/M does not.

16. It now seems reasonable to suggest that genes that play a key role in some environments will in some sense simply cease to exist as genes—never be transcribed—in others. Insofar as what it means to be a gene as opposed to a stretch of noncoding DNA is that that stretch or those related stretches of DNA actually code for some protein or other, or play some role in genetic control (i.e., gene regulation) at other levels, I do not think it is at all at odds with our current knowledge of gene-environment and gene-gene interactions to suggest that in some environments, areas that code in other environments simply won't code for anything at all—will never be "read," or at least never be read as a gene. Certainly, gene-regulation in developmental biology points toward the importance of the environment in "deciding" which genes will be read; this might, for example, be the result of phenotypic plasticity at the level of "regulatory plasticity" (see Schlichting and Pigliucci 1998, 72ff.). Fausto-Sterling explores a similar topic, the way that taking a "reaction-norm" perspective can radically alter the way one views the relationship between a particular biological finding and an associated behavior, in her "Beyond Difference: A Biologist's Perspective" (1997, see esp. 245–49). To follow this up, however, would take us rather too far afield.

Faderman, making a related point, suggests several hypothetical ways in which biological correlates to homosexuality could be expressed as a tendency toward homosexual identity only within some cultural contexts and not others, as the way that one's own sexuality is perceived is modified by cultural expectations (1994, 13–14).

17. Hamer, apparently, actually tried to find a correlation; dividing gay sib-pairs into those that were concordant for their Xq28 markers and those that were discordant, he tried to find a difference in correlation between preferred sexual activities (and specifically, between those who listed "receptive anal intercourse" as their preferred sexual activity). No such correlation was to be found, and Hamer concludes that "there is as yet no evidence that the particular sexual activity a person prefers is genetically influenced." Hamer and Copeland 1994, 168–69.

18. Murphy argues that much research into sexuality and sexual orientation is valuable, something I do not deny at all. The research that Murphy suggests as very useful (for example, specific health risks and problems, or research into parenting success as a way of arguing specific legal cases, etc.) may well be useful and valuable. However, again, I do not believe that at this time research into the etiologies of orientation could be better than useless, as they are likely to be dangerously mis- and overinterpreted.

Chapter 7

1. Many researchers cite Kagan's work on the heritability of temperament as very convincing, but have problems with some of the claimed physiological correlations. Hamer and Copeland, for example, while praising Kagan's work in general, think that many of his correlations— especially those involve eye and skin color—are likely spurious. They note that while some of the physiological correlations have been replicated, "eye color" has not been, and that the story to account for it was "spun out of thin air" (Hamer and Copeland 1998, 65).

2. For an interesting analysis of how depression, and mental illness in general, gets created as a form of "brain dysfunction" see Szasz (1987).

3. But see Kramer (1993) on the increased confidence that often comes with the successful treatment of depression, and on the way in which this confidence can be translated into a willingness to change environments (see esp. 271–72).

4. Especially since, given the near-ubiquity of drug-based treatments in all modern institutional settings, these data come primarily from the mostly truly horrible institutions that existed before the rise of medical approaches to mental illness. See, for example, MacDonald's description of "institutions" for the mad in *Mystical Bedlam* (1981).

5. This is related to Dobzhansky's comment that gaining "complete knowledge of a norm of reaction" is a "practical impossibility" because "the performance of a genotype cannot be tested in all possible environments" as "the latter are infinitely variable" and in any event "new environments are constantly produced" (Dobzhansky 1955, 74–77). See also Platt and Bach 1997, 137–38.

6. See Foucault's "The Politics of Health in the Eighteenth Century" for further discussion of these issues, and note that the move from hygiene education to vaccination programs was another stabilizing move, both politically and socially. A vaccination program does not even broach the question of the availability of the necessities of basic hygiene, of the sorts of living conditions the lower classes were (and still are) forced into, whereas hygiene education would (and to some extent did) force the state to deal with these issues.

   Consider another example. Lewontin notes that the high death rate from tuberculosis in the nineteenth century was at least in part the result of poor living and working conditions that both fostered its spread and made it a much more dangerous disease. In a different environment, treating tuberculosis would be for the most part irrelevant, since it would cease to be a problem (Lewontin 1993, 41–43). Currently, we are faced with the recreation of the sorts of abysmal living conditions that create the right opportunities for the rapid spread of tuberculosis (high concentrations of people with immune systems weakened from everything from exposure, poor diets, and immunosuppressive diseases) and once again tuberculosis has become problematic, with the creation and spread of multiply antibiotic resistant strains. The treatment of tuberculosis as an internal relationship between a bacterium and a person has the effect of hiding the significance of its reemergence, and prevents the questioning of a society that allows a significant portion of its population to go hungry, without shelter, and without adequate medical treatment, the preconditions necessary for such a reemergence.

It is interesting in this context to note that the *danger* of TB's reemergence is said to come from the multiply antibiotic-resistant nature of some of the strains, and that this is blamed primarily not on the overprescription of antibiotics, nor on the medical community's blind trust in antibiotics having permitted it to ignore the conditions necessary for a disease such as TB to spread, but rather on *patients* not finishing their antibiotic sequences. Once again, the problem is made out to be internal to the patients, and the social conditions necessary for the creation and spread of new antibiotic-resistant strains are ignored. For example, this analysis ignores the way in which the move to highly superficial and high-speed doctor-patient relationships made, for many people, understanding their doctors' instructions problematic. It ignored the way that the lack of availability of primary care and hence the reliance in low-income communities of getting primary health care through emergency rooms results in particularly cursory explanations. It ignores the way in which the medical community, in considering the treatment of low-income patients a somewhat secondary concern and taking an authoritative approach to medicine in low-income communities, created a severe loss of doctor-patient trust, and the way that this lack of trust is translated into an unwillingness to follow instructions.

Chapter 8

1. On this topic, see Klein's brilliant "postmodern diet book," *Eat Fat*, in which he "aims to recall" the beauty of fat against the cultural obsession with thin (Klein 1996, preface).

2. The breakdown is as follows: "Type I is characterized by excess total body fat without any particular concentration of fat in a given area of the body. . . . Type II is defined as excess subcutaneous fat on the trunk, particularly in the abdominal area, and is equivalent to the so-called android or male type of fat deposition. Type III is characterized by and excessive amount of fat in the abdominal visceral area and can be labeled abdominal visceral obesity. The last type (type IV) is defined as gluteo-femoral obesity and is observed primarily in women (gynoid obesity)." (Bouchard and Pérusse 1993, 26). It should be noted that, along with different correlations between BMIs and body fat percentages for different ethnicities, variations in where the fat is carried are statistically correlated with different ethnicities as well. See esp. Duncan et al. 1995 and Ortiz et al. 1992.

3. I hint at another possible interpretation of these results below; namely, that the correlation that moderate obesity has with increased health risks is at least in part explicable by the correlation it has with weight cycling and dieting, both of which may be associated with increased health risks independent of absolute weight or body fat percentages. Due to the paucity of research on this topic, though, this remains, for the moment, speculative.

4. This is excepting those cases where there is an obvious metabolic disorder that is genetic in origin. These cases, however, are not in any event constitutive of the heritability estimates of obesity.

Chapter 9

1. Another worrisome aspect, and one that might be thought to follow more from this culture's extreme gender inequalities rather than from the genetic as defining parenthood *simpliciter*, is that the emphasis on the genetic as defining parenthood tends to discount women's gestational contribution (at least as far as rights are concerned), both to the developmental process narrowly construed, and in terms of the actual labor, time commitment,

and the like, involved in bearing a child. Since this cultural emphasis on the genetic does not extend to limiting women's responsibility for the "purity" of the gestational environment during pregnancy, the control of women's bodies during pregnancy is decoupled from "motherhood," that is, from specifically parental rights and responsibilities. In other words, what grants the rights associated with motherhood becomes the genetic; however, the responsibility for maintaining a "pure" gestational environment can only rest with the gestational mother. If those tasks thought necessary to ensure having a "healthy" baby are no longer those associated with the legal status of being a mother, the task of insuring fetal health becomes a responsibility dissociated from *parental* rights and responsibilities. As we shall see, in the case of pregnancy contracts where in vitro fertilization (IVF) is used, this makes the gestational mother out to be a nonmother who yet has vast responsibilities in terms of ensuring fetal health. The only relationship she is supposed to have with the fetus is one construed entirely in terms of producing a product—a healthy baby. Insofar as this decoupling tends toward a commodification of gestational labor in these cases (but in such a way that the reasoning can be extended more generally), the control of women's bodies during pregnancy for the sake of a product in which the gestational relationship is thought to contribute nothing beyond the formation of a commodity is made particularly disturbing. However interesting this line of reasoning may be, following it up would take us too far afield of the major focus of this chapter. For a different view of the causal history of control of women's bodies during pregnancy, see Morris 1997.

2. Throughout this chapter, I will speak of "parental rights" in a rather cavalier way. I do not mean by this, however, to support any particular notion of "parental rights" nor to imply that parents should have any rights qua parents. On this very interesting topic see Dwyer 1995 and 1998.

3. See, for example, *In the Matter of Baby M* (109 N.J. 537 A.2d [Atlantic Reporter, 2d series] 1227, see esp. 1234–35) (court finds the contract "illegal" and "void"); *Matter of Adoption of Baby Girl L.J.* (N.Y.S., 505 N.Y.S.2d 813) (court finds the contract not necessarily illegal and void, but rather "voidable"); *Matter of Adoption of Paul* (N.Y.S., 550 N.Y.S2d 815) (court finds, contra decision in *Baby Girl L.J.* case, contract void and explicitly states that any payment is illegal); *Doe v. Kelley* (Mich.App., 307 N.W.2d 438) (court finds that pregnancy contracts are illegal, and denies the applicability of the privacy right re: procreation to the case); *Surrogate Patenting Assocs. v. Kentucky* (704 S.W.2d 209), cited above (court affirms the in principle legality of pregnancy contracts, including those for money, but maintains that they are still "voidable" by the "surrogate" mother), *In Re Marriage of Cynthia J.* (25 Cal. App. 4th 1218) (court finds that the contract is unenforceable). See Ellman et al. 1991, 1322–23 for summaries of some of these cases. In any event, as Ellman et al. 1991 points out, there has been no case pertaining to contract pregnancies where the so-called surrogate was both the gestational and the genetic mother where the courts have found that the *contract* is even relevant to "compelling an unwilling surrogate mother [sic] to surrender her child" (Ellman et al. 1991, 1322).

4. I am uncomfortable with the phrase "genetic mother" and believe it to be misleading in an important way. Where the "gestational" and "genetic" mothers are pulled apart (in the cases discussed next), what the "genetic" mother contributes is not merely half a human genome, nor is the rest of the egg simply raw material in any sense of the words. Rather, it is a cell of significant complexity, without whose proteins, enzymes, and the like the half-genome that each genetic parent contributes would be entirely useless. In referring to, for example, egg donors as "genetic mothers" one ignores the significant nongenetic (and perhaps non-nuclear genetic) role that the egg plays. This includes, for example, not only carrying all the proteins and enzymes necessary for DNA and cellular replication, but also carrying all the mitochondria (and other organelles and subcellular "machinery"), along with all the mitochondrial DNA. This pretends, falsely and perniciously, that the egg and the sperm represent a roughly equal contribution from the standpoint of developmental biology.

Calling the woman who contributes the egg a *genetic* mother and putting her contribution in terms of the genetic material, is obviously a move that makes what men contribute and what women contribute to pregnancies seem at least potentially equal, in a way that strikes me as false.

5. The number of possible "parents" in these cases can grow quite rapidly. Usually, it is claimed that there can be five possible "parents"—the genetic mother, the genetic father, the gestational mother, the "social" or "functional" mother (she who will raise the child), and the "social" or "functional" father (he who will raise the child) (see for example Pierce-Gealy 1995, 542; Hill 1991, 355). Given the "intent" doctrine articulated in the *Johnson v. Calvert* case, we might think that there is even room for some number of participants who *initiate* the process and *cause* (in a historical sense) the child to be born. Were the possibility of multiple-parenting arrangements and shared custody issues are taken into account, of course, the numbers would become even larger. Hill lists sixteen different possible reproductive methods, based on the source of the gametes, the site of fertilization, and the site of the pregnancy (Hill 1991, 542), some of which have never been used (and, given their baroqueness, probably never will be used). Below, at note 16, I note some other possibilities that new technologies might create.

6. As will be discussed below, there are two other relevant cases. In one there was no conflict of any sort between the participants in the case, and in the other there was a custody battle between the gestational but not genetic mother and the father to whom she had been married prior to a divorce.

7. Interestingly, in *Belsito v. Clark* (discussed in detail below) the judge also noted that proof of giving birth used to be an acceptable proof of being a "natural" parent because "for millennia, giving birth was synonymous with providing the genetic makeup of the child that was born" (*Belsito v. Clark*, 67 Ohio Misc. 2d 54)—that is, was proof of the existence of the more fundamental "blood" relationship.

8. In her "Surrogacy, Slavery, and African-American Women" (written before the California Supreme Court decision) Allen raised the same objection to what she saw as the likely outcome of *Johnson v. Calvert* (a court decision affirming intention as the important deciding factor), and also suggested that the child's best interest be used instead, just as in "ordinary" custody battles (Allen 1991, 25). However, as above, and as Allen notes, this will often have the effect of putting so-called surrogates in a position where they are, if not certain to lose, at least quite likely to lose (they, after all, are almost always financially less well off) (Allen 1991, 26). As Allen points out, the situation is made worse in gestational mothers who give birth to children of a different race, as courts are likely to treat multiracial families as problematic (Allen1991, 29–30).

9. As is often the case in surrogate arrangements, Carol and Shelly were related. Specifically, they were sisters. So in this case, it turns out that it is *not* true that Nicholas (the resulting child) was not particularly closely genetically related to Carol, as Carol was his maternal aunt.

10. Eastman argues that this is nothing more than a "veiled" intent standard, since if one consents to waive one's rights, one is not intending to create and raise the child, and if one is so intending, than one will not, presumably, waive one's rights (1995, 555).

11. See Ellman et al. 1991 1323 and Corea 1985, chapter 3; see also Ellman et al. 1991, s883–85, on the Uniform Parentage Act (but see below on its more recent restrictions). While the UPA was meant to make state laws consistent on issues of parentage, different states have enacted it in slightly different versions (see 9A West's U.Laws Ann. 593, 1985 supp. p. 311). These differences with respect to the treatment of children from cases of artificial insemination by donor when performed by a physician are not, however, significant.

12. See for example Ellman et al. 1991, 938ff., and its discussion of *Michael H. v. Gerald D.* (109

S. Ct. 2333, 1989), especially 956–60. Note especially the new California law mentioned, which allows a man "to move for blood testing to establish paternity, even though the mother is married to another man, if the motion is made within two years of the child's birth" (*Michael H. v. Gerald D.*, 959). While not explicitly mentioned, it is hard to see how the scope of this would not encompass at least many AID cases as well.

13. Any full analysis of the issues surrounding contract pregnancies would have to include an analysis of the idea that people "own" their genes (and, e.g., tissue) in a sense that grants them something like property rights (see the quotes by Gilbert, above). The law in this area, though, is very unsettled. As we do not think of parents as "owning" their children, it is unclear what force the ownership claim surrounding one's own DNA is supposed to have with respect to parental rights. The complexities of the issues forbid an exploration of them here, and to follow up this topic would take us too far afield.

14. For more on this topic, see chapter 10. See also the growing body of work on "developmental systems theory," and approaches to developmental biology more generally that attempts to free it from the privileging of the genetic over other aspects of developmental biology (see for example Griffiths and Gray 1994; Johnston and Gottlieb 1990; Oyama 1985; and citations therein).

15. One might think it hard to reconcile this stand with the bold statement that "under Ohio law, when a child is delivered by a gestational surrogate who has been impregnated through the process of in vitro fertilization, the natural parents of the child be identified by a determination as to which individuals have provided the genetic imprint for that child" (66). However, recall that the judge in this case separated out the concept of a "natural" parent from the parent who gets the rights and responsibilities of parenthood (a legal parent). The genetic parents would *definitely* be the natural parents, the judge seems to be saying, but "a genetic test cannot be the only basis for determining who will assume the status of legal parent" (66). However, it seems likely that being declared the "natural parent" as a matter of law would help in a custody battle.

16. Future reproductive technologies may provide even more "options." For example, "adult" cloning would permit there to be only one genetic parent, moving DNA from eggs into sperm would permit there to be two genetic mothers, moving DNA from sperm into eggs would permit two genetic fathers and a partial genetic mother—the woman who donated the egg would still be genetically related to the resulting child with respect to the non-nuclear (mitochondrial) DNA, so there would be three genetic parents.

17. See for example Wittgenstein's *Remarks on Frazer's Golden Bough* for an interesting discussion of interpreting early anthropological reports. More prosaically, early anthropological reports often underestimate the sophistication of the respondents' beliefs.

18. The case of children being brought up by homosexual couples is a case in point here. A narrow "best interest" clause might be interpreted by conservative courts to point away from giving custody to homosexual parents in these cases,—if not on any stand against homosexuality qua homosexuality, then perhaps on some more nebulous grounds. Certainly the history of the courts in this context is not encouraging. See Ellman et al. 1991, 517–29. In this context, the cases of *Jarrett v. Jarrett* (mother loses custody based on court's determination that her "cohabiting" with a man with whom she was not married creates "moral hazards" for her children, and may put them in awkward situations when they are "compelled to try to explain [the man with whom their mother was living]'s presence to their friends," Ellman et al. 1991, 517–21) and *Roe v. Roe* (father loses custody based on court's determination that his engaging in homosexual relationships made him an unfit father, and that the child's best interest were served by granting the mother sole custody, Ellman et al. 1991, 521–23), are especially troubling.

Chapter 10

1. A similar point is made by Longino; see especially chapters 6 and 7 of her *Science as Social Knowledge* (1990).

2. This is obviously part of a more general and complex critique of the relationship between the way the world is conceptualized/categorized and social/political issues. Obviously, though, following this up would take us rather far afield, and would be a significant project in and of itself. But see for example Dupré 1993, Longino 1990, and MacKinnon 1984.

3. This may be linked to a more general problem with a similar "habit of thought" in evolutionary biology discussed above. On a view that makes the organism out to be separable from the environment in the way described above, "fitness" (on whatever interpretation) ends up residing entirely in the organism (narrowly construed). There is a firm line conceived between the organism and the world, and while it is always admitted that that line can be and is often crossed, that very conception may well be implicated in a habit of thought that results in an asymmetrical conception of the way environments and organisms interact. See Oyama 1985 for discussion and critique of the way these sorts of habits of thought influence research.

4. Although it will also emerge below that the claims I am citing to support my contention that many researchers assume environmental stability may be claims by the researchers that their research has *shown* that the environment will be stable in some sense; that is, the claim may be that the research supports the claim, not that it is supported by the claim. In any event, unless very strong assumptions are made about the additive nature of the genotype-environment interactions or insensitivity of the genotypes to the environments in question, some assumptions about environmental stability must be used to get the research off the ground. More on this below.

5. It is odd, and somewhat suspicious, that for some reason in these contexts this principle is often phrased in such a way that it makes it look as if it is only the attempt to increase the well-being of those less well-off now that generates the zero-sum problems; making the well-off even better off is rarely mentioned, let alone assumed to be equally problematic.

6. Lest the reader think I am unfairly maligning Herrnstein and Murray, I will quote a few relevant passages at length:

    The same burden of complications that are only a nuisance to people who are smart enough are much more of a barrier to people who are not. . . . [In the past] you could get ahead by hard work. No one would stand in your way. Today that is no longer true. American society has erected barriers to individual sweat equity. . . . Credentialism is a closely related problem. . . . Increasingly, occupations must be licenced . . . but the benefits [of licensing] are often outweighed by the costs of the increased bureaucratization . . . (1994, 542).

    Imagine living in a society where the rules about crime are simple and the consequences are equally simple. "Crime" consists of a few obviously wrong acts. . . . Someone who commits a crime is probably caught, and almost certainly punished. . . . Punishment . . . is meaningful [and] follows arrest quickly. . . . Living in such a world, the moral compass shows simple, easily understood directions. North is north, south is south, right is right, and wrong is wrong.

    Now imagine that all the rules are made more complicated. The number of acts defined as crimes has multiplied. . . . The link between moral transgression and committing crime is made harder to understand. . . . To top it all off, even the "wrongness" of the basic crimes is called into question. . . .

    The two worlds we have described are not far removed from the contrast between the criminal justice system in the United States as recently as the 1950s and that system as of the 1990s (1994, 543–44).

I am utterly unable to fathom how Herrnstein and Murray could have written the above, apparently in all seriousness. Apparently, and as usual, they are thinking of the sorts of laws that matter to them—contract, stock trading, etc. But the number of "victimless" crimes that were on the books in the 1950s, and the treatment that, for example, homosexuals received then, is utterly appalling; the criminal justice system's treatment of black Americans in the 1950s horrific even by today's rather low standards. Their faith that a more free-market attitude will result in the poor being better off would be touching if it didn't come across as so blatantly disingenuous. They do not, for example, ever suggest that the doctors who treat them and the lawyers who represent them (as members of the upper middle class) shouldn't be licensed.

7. Plants that show significant phenotypic plasticity may also "choose" what environment they are exposed to, by for example concentrating on vertical growth to avoid shade from competitors (see for example Schlichting and Pigliucci 1998).

8. Our ability to influence, albeit somewhat indirectly and in an unguided fashion, long-term climatic changes, for example, makes it seem somewhat unlikely that any changes in the environment are completely isolated from human influence. Certain geological phenomena (plate tectonics?) may be the best candidates.

9. This once again brings up the interesting issue of how to think about genes for a trait in environments in which that trait is (deeply) irrelevant. (E.g., if they are no longer influencing that trait, what are they influencing? Do they necessarily code for anything at all? And if not, should they still be thought of as genes, and if so, as genes for what? And so on.) See discussion in chapter 6.

10. For some examples of such research programs, see Schlichting and Pigliucci 1998; Pigliucci and Schlichting 1997; Griffiths and Gray 1994; various in Griffiths, ed., 1992; Johnston and Gottlieb 1990; Odling-Smee 1988; Plotkin 1988; Levins and Lewontin 1985; and Oyama 1985.

REFERENCES

Acuff, K. L. and R. R. Faden, 1991. "A History of Prenatal and Newborn Screening Programs: Lessons for the Future," in R. Faden, G. Geller, M. Powers, eds., *AIDS, Women, and the Next Generation*, New York, Oxford University Press, 58–93.

Aldhous, P. 1992: "The Promise and Pitfalls of Molecular Genetics." *Science* 257, 164.

Allen, A. 1988. "Privacy, Surrogacy, and the *Baby M* Case." *Georgetown Law Journal* 76, 1759–92.

———. 1990. "Surrogacy, Slavery, and the Ownership of Life." *Harvard Journal of Law and Public Policy* 13, 139–49.

———. 1991. "Surrogacy, Slavery, and African-American Women." Draft, Lott Manuscript.

Allison, D. B., S. Heshka, M. C. Neale, D. T. Lykken, and S. B. Heymsfield. 1994. "A Genetic Analysis of Relative Weight among 4,020 Twin Pairs, with an Emphasis on Sex Effects." *Health Psychology* 13(4), 362–65.

Allison, D. B., J. Kaprio, M. Korkeila, M. Koshenvuo, M. C. Neale, and K. Hayakaway. 1996. "The Heritability of Body Mass Index among an International Sample of Monozygotic Twins Reared Apart." *International Journal of Obesity Related Metabolic Disorders* 20(6), 501–6.

Altenberg L. and Wagner G. P. 1996. "Complex Adaptations and the Evolution of Evolvability." *Evolution* 50(3), 967–76.

American Academy of Pediatrics (Committee on Genetics, Desposito et al.). 1996. "Newborn Screening Fact Sheet." *Pediatrics* 98, 473–501.

Angier, N. 1996a. "People Haunted by Anxiety Appear to Be Short on a Gene." *New York Times*, November 29, 1996, sec. A, p. 1, col. 5.

———. 1996b. "Variant Gene Tied to a Love of New Thrills," *New York Times*, January 2, 1996, sec. A, p. 1, col. 1.

Annas, G. J. 1991. "Crazy Making: Embryos and Gestational Mothers." *Hastings Center Report* 21, 35.

Appiah, K. A. 1994. "Identity, Authenticity, Survival: Multicultural Societies and Social Reproduction." In *Multiculturalism: Examining the Politics of Recognition*, edited by A. Gutmann. Princeton, N.J.: Princeton University Press.

Arneson, R. J. 1992. "Commodification and Commercial Surrogacy." *Philosophy and Public Affairs* 21(2) (Spring), 132–64.

Arvey, R. D., B. P. McCall, T. J. Bouchard Jr., P. Taubman, and M. A. Cavanaugh. 1994. "Genetic Influences on Job Satisfaction and Work Values." *Personality and Individual Difference* 17(1), 21–33.

Associated Press. 1997. "Gene Discovery May Yield Test for Glaucoma." *New York Times*, January 31, 1997, sec. A, p. 15, col. 1.

Avigad, S., S. Kleiman, M. Weinstein, B. E. Cohen, G. Schwartz, S. L. Woo, and Y. Shiloh.

1991. "Compound Heterozygosity in Nonphenylketonuria Hyperphenylalanemia: The Contributions of Mutations for Classical Phenylketonuria." *American Journal of Human Genetics* 49(2) (August), 393–99.

Bailey, J. M. and A. P. Bell. 1993. "Familiality of Female and Male Homosexuality." *Behavior Genetics* 23(4), 313–22.

Bailey, R. C. 1997: "Hereditarian Scientific Fallacies." *Genetica* 99, 125–33.

Barinaga, M. 1995. "'Obese' Protein Slims Mice." *Science* 269, 475–76.

———. 1996. "Obesity: Leptin Receptor Weighs In." *Science* 271, 29.

Baron, M. 1997. "Genetic Linkage and Biopolar Mood Affective Disorder: Progress and Pitfalls." *Molecular Psychiatry* 2, 100–210.

Bartholet, E. 1993. *Family Bonds: Adoption and the Politics of Parenting.* New York: Houghton Mifflin.

Behne, A. 1996–97. "Balancing the Adoption Triangle: The State, the Adoptive Parents, and the Birth Parents—Where Does the Adoptee Fit In?" *Buffalo Journal of Public Interest Law* 15, 49–83.

Bem, D. J. 1996. "Exotic Becomes Erotic: A Political Postscript".

Berman, J. L., G. C. Cunningham, R. W. Day, R. Ford, and D. Y. Y. Hsia. 1969. "Causes for High Phenylalanine with Normal Tyrosine," *American Journal of Diseases of Children* 117, 54–65.

Beumont, P. J. V. 1988. "Obesity as Human Predicament." In *Handbook of Eating Disorders, Part 2: Obesity,* edited by G. D. Burrows, P. J. V. Beumont, and R. C. Casper. New York: Elsevier.

Blakeslee, S. 1996. "Researchers Track Down a Gene That May Govern Spatial Abilities." *New York Times,* July 23, 1996, sec. C; p. 3; col. 4.

Block, N. 1995. "How Heritability Misleads about Race." *Cognition* 56, 90–128.

Bouchard, C. 1997. "Genetics of Human Obesity: Recent Results from Linkage Studies." *Journal of Nutrition* 127, 1887S–1890S.

Bouchard, C. and L. Pérusse. 1993. "Genetic Aspects of Obesity." In *Annals of the New York Academy of Sciences* 699 (October 29), *Prevention and Treatment of Childhood Obesity,* edited by C. L. Williams and S. Y. S. Kimm. New York: New York Academy of Sciences.

Bouchard, T. J., D. L. Lykken, M. McGrue, N. L. Segal, and A. Tellegenet. 1990. "Sources of Human Psychological Difference: The Minnesota Twin Study of Twins Reared Apart," *Science* 250, 4978.

———. 1994. "Sources of Human Psychological Differences: The Minnesota Study of Twins Reared Apart," *Science* 250, 223–28.

Brandon, R. N., 1990. *Adaptation and Environment.* Princeton, N.J.: Princeton University Press.

Bray, G. A. 1987. "Overweight Is Risking Fate: Definition, Classification, Prevalence, and Risks." In *Annals of the New York Academy of Sciences* 499 (June 15), *Human Obesity,* edited by R. J. Wurtman and J. J. Wurtman. New York: New York Academy of Sciences.

Brinster, R. L. and J. Zimmerman, 1994. "Spermatogenesis Following Male Germ-cell Transplantation," *Proceedings of the National Academy of Sciences of the United States of America* 91(24), 11298–302.

Brown, P. J., and M. Konner. 1987. "An Anthropological Perspective on Obesity." In *Annals of the New York Academy of Sciences* 499 (June 15) *Human Obesity,* edited by R. J. Wurtman and J. J. Wurtman. New York: New York Academy of Sciences.

Brownell, K. D. 1991. "Dieting and the Search for the Perfect Body." *Behavior Therapy* 22, 1–12.

Brownell, K. D. and T. A. Wadden. 1991. "The Heterogeneity of Obesity: Fitting Treatments to Individuals," *Behavior Therapy* 22, 153–77.

Brunner, H. G., M. Nelen, X. O. Breakefield, H. H. Ropers, and B. A. Van Oost. 1993. "Abnormal Behavior Associated with a Point Mutation in the Structural Gene for Monoamine Oxidase A." *Science* 262, 578–80.

Burns, G. W. 1983. *The Science of Genetics: An Introduction to Heredity.* New York: Macmillan.

Buss, D. 1994. *The Evolution of Desire.* New York: Basic Books.

Butler, J. 1993. *Bodies That Matter.* New York: Routledge.

Campfield, L. A., F. J. Smith, Y. Guisez, R. Devos, and P. Burn. 1995. "Recombinant Mouse OB Protein: Evidence for a Peripheral Signal Linking Adiposity and Central Neural Networks." *Science* 269, 546–49.

Canguilhem, G. 1991. *The Normal and the Pathological.* New York: Zone Books.

Cantor, C. 1992. "The Challenges to Technology and Informatics." In D. J. Kevles and L. Hood, eds., *The Code of Codes: Scientific and Social Issues in the Human Genome Project.* Cambridge, Mass.: Harvard University Press, 98–111.

Caplan, A. L., H. T. Engelhardt, Jr., and J. J. McCartney (eds.), 1981. *Concepts of Health and Disease: Interdisciplinary Perspectives.* Reading, Mass.: Addison-Wesley, Advanced Book Program.

Carrier, J. M. 1976. "Cultural Factors Affecting Urban Mexican Male Homosexual Behavior." *Archives of Sexual Behavior* 5(2), 103–24.

Carey, G. and D. L. DiLalla. 1994. "Personality and Psychopathology: Genetic Perspectives," *Journal of Abnormal Psychology* 103(1), 32–43.

Caskey, C. T. 1992. "DNA-Based Medicine: Prevention and Therapy." In D. J. Kevles and L. Hood, eds., *The Code of Codes: Scientific and Social Issues in the Human Genome Project.* Cambridge, Mass.: Harvard University Press.

Cavalli-Sforza, L. L. and F. Cavalli-Sforza. 1995. *The Great Human Diasporas.* Reading, Mass.: Helix Books.

Chorney, M. J., J. Chorney, N. Seese, M. J. Owen, J. Daniels, P. McGuffin, L. A. Thompson, D. K. Detterman, C. Benbow, D. Lubinski, T. Eley, and R. Plomin. 1998. "A Quantitative Trait Locus Associated with Cognitive Ability in Children." *Psychological-Science* 9(3), 159–66.

Clark, L. A., D. Watson, and S. Mineka. 1994. "Temperament, Personality, and the Mood and Anxiety Disorders." *Journal of Abnormal Psychology* 103, 103–16.

Coleman, M. 1996. "Gestation, Intent and the Seed: Defining Motherhood in the Era of Assisted Human Reproduction." *Cardozo Law Review* 17, 497–530.

Collins, F. 1989. *Human Genome Initiative.* Hearing before the Subcommittee on Science, Technology, and Space, of the Committee on Commerce, Science and Transportation, United States Senate, One Hundred First Congress, First Session on The Human Genome Initiative and the Future of Biotechnology, Nov. 9, 1989.

Connolly, H. M., J. L. Crary, M. D. McGoon, D. D.Hensrud, B. S. Edwards, W. D. Edwards, and H. V. Schaff. 1997. "Valvular Heart Disease Associated with Fenfluramine-Phentermine." *New England Journal of Medine* 337, 581–88.

Considine, R. V., M. K. Sinha, M. L. Heiman, A. Krianuciunas, T. W. Stephens, M. R. Nyce, J. P. Ohannesian, C. C. Marco, L. J. McKee, and T. L. Bauer, et al. 1996. "Serum Immunoreactive-Leptin Concentrations in Normal-Weight and Obese Humans." *New England Journal of Medicine* 334(5). 324–25.

Cooper, R. M. and J. P. Zubek. 1958. "Effects of Enriched and Restricted Early Environments on the Learning Ability of Bright and Dull Rats." *Canadian Journal of Psychology* 12, 159–64.

Corea, G. 1985. *The Mother Machine.* New York: Harper & Row.

Craddock, D. 1988. "Obesity in General Practice." In *Handbook of Eating Disorders, Part 2: Obesity,* edited by G. D. Burrows, P. J. V. Beumont, and R. C. Casper. New York: Elsevier.

Crittenden, D. 1995. "Yes, Motherhood Lowers Pay." *New York Times,* August 22, 1995, Op-Ed, sec. A, p. 11.

Cropanzano, R., and K. James. 1990. "Some Methodological Considerations for the Behavioral Genetic Analysis of Work Attitudes." *Journal of Applied Psychology* 75(4), 433–39.

Crow, J. F. 1986. *Basic Concepts in Population, Quantitative, and Evolutionary Genetics.* New York: W. H. Freeman and Company.

Daniels, J., P. McGuffin, and M. Owen. 1996. "Molecular Genetic Research on IQ: Can It Be Done? Should It Be Done?" *Journal of BioSocial Science* 28, 491–507.

Davis, J. O., J. A. Phelps, and H. S. Bracha. 1995. "Prenatal Development of Monozygotic Twins and Concordance for Schizoprenia." *Schizophrenia Bulletin* 21(3), 357–66.

Dawkins, R. 1976. *The Selfish Gene.* New York: Oxford University Press.

———. 1981. "Selfish Genes in Race or Politics." *Nature* 289, 528.

———. 1982. *The Extended Phenotype.* New York: W. H. Freeman and Company.

———. 1986. *The Blind Watchmaker.* New York: Oxford University Press.

Després, J. P., S. Moorjani, P. J. Lupien, A. Tremblay, A. Nadeau, and C. Bouchard. 1992. "Genetic Aspects of Susceptibility to Obesity and Related Dyslipidemias." *Molecular and Cellular Biochemistry* 113, 151–69.

de Vos, G. 1992. *Social Cohesion and Alienation: Minorities in the United States and Japan.* Boulder, Colo.: Westview Press.

DiLalla, L. F. and I. I. Gottesman. 1991. "Biological and Genetic Contributors to Violence— Widom's Untold Tale." *Psychological Bulletin* 109(1), 125–29.

Dion, K. K. and S. Stein. 1978. "Physical Attractiveness and Interpersonal Influence." *Journal of Experimental Social Psychology* 14, 97–108.

Dion, K. L., and K. K. Dion. 1987. "Belief in a Just World and Physical Attractiveness Stereotyping." *Journal of Personality and Social Psychology* 52(4), 775–80.

Dobzhansky, T. 1955. *Evolution, Genetics, and Man.* New York: John Wiley and Sons.

Dobzhansky, T., and B. Spassky. 1944. "Genetics of Natural Populations. XI. Manifestation of Genetic Variants in *Drosophila pseudoobscura* in Different Environments," *Genetics* 29, 270– 90. Reprinted in *Dobzhansky's Genetics of Natural Populations: I–XLIII*, edited by R. C. Lewontin, J. A. Moore, W. B. Provine, and B. Wallace. New York: Columbia University Press, 1981.

Duncan, D. D., L. E. Chambless, M. I. Schmidt, M. Szklo, A. R. Folsom, M. A. Carpenter, and J. R. Crouse III. 1995. "Correlates of Body Fat Distribution: Variation across Categories of Race, Sex, and Body Mass in the Atherosclerosis Risk in Communities Study." *Annals of Epidemiology* 5(3), 192–200.

Dupré, J. 1993. *The Disorder of Things.* Cambridge, Mass.: Harvard University Press.

———. 1997. "Sociobiology Redux: Recent Speculations on the Biology of Gender." Manuscript presented at the Jing Lyman Lecture Series, Stanford University..

Dwyer, J. G. 1995. "Religious Schooling in a Liberal Society: Parents' Rights, Community Rights, and Justice for Children." Doctoral dissertation, Stanford University Philosophy Department.

———. 1998. *Religious Schools v. Children's Rights.* Ithaca, N.Y.: Cornell University Press.

Eisensmith, R. C., D. R. Martinez, A. I. Kuzmin, A. A. Goltsov, A. Brown, R. Singh, L. F. Elsas II, S. W. Woo, 1996. "Molecular Basis of Phenylketonuria and a Correlation between Genotype and Phenotype in a Heterogeneous Southeastern US Population," *Pediatrics* 97(4), 512–16.

Ellman, I. M., P. M. Kurtz, and K. T. Bartlett, eds. 1991. *Family Law: Cases, Text, Problems.* 2nd ed. Charlottesville, Va.: The Michie Company.

Ernulf, K. E., S. M. Innala, and F. L. Whitam. 1989. "Biological Explanation, Psychological Explanation, and Tolerance of Homosexuals: A Cross-National Analysis of Beliefs and Attitudes. *Psychological Reports* 65, 1003–10.

Faderman, L. 1981. *Surpassing the Love of Men: Romantic Friendship and Love between Women from the Renaissance to the Present.* New York: Quill, William Morrow.

———. 1994. "The Social Construction of Lesbianism: Address to the *American Psychological Association, Division 44.* August 14, 1994. Draft.

Fausto-Sterling, A. 1985. *Myths of Gender.* New York: Basic Books.

———. 1997. "Beyond Difference: A Biologist's Perspective." *Journal of Social Issues* 53(2), 233– 58.

Feldman, M., and R. C. Lewontin, 1975. "The Heritability Hangup," *Science* 190, 1163–68.

Fölling, I. 1994. "The Discovery of Phenylketonuria." *Acta Paediatrics Supplement* 407, 4–10.

Foucault, M. 1976. "The Politics of Health in the Eighteenth Century," reprinted in *Power/ Knowledge* (1980), ed.and trans. C. Gordon. New York: Pantheon Books.

———. 1978. *The History of Sexuality, Volume 1: An Introduction,* translated by R. Hurley. New York: Vintage.

————. 1985. *The History of Sexuality, Volume 2: The Use of Pleasure,* translated by R. Hurley. New York: Vintage.

Gaudio, R. P. 1994. "Sounding Gay: Pitch Properties in the Speech of Gay and Straight Men." *American Speech* 69(1), 30–57.

Gibbs, W. W. 1995 "Seeking the Criminal Element." *Scientific American,* March 1995, 100–107.

Gilbert, W. 1992. "A Vision of the Grail." In D. J. Kevles and L. Hood, eds., *The Code of Codes: Scientific and Social Issues in the Human Genome Project.* Cambridge, Mass.: Harvard University Press.

Goodhart, C. 1994. "Does a Brighter Future Beckon? Our Genetic Inheritance Should Influence Educational Policy." *New Scientist,* October 22, Forum, 50.

Gottlied, K., and D. K. Manchester. 1986. "Twin Study Methodology and Variability in Xenobiotic Placental Metabolism." *Teratogenesis Carcinogenesis and Mutagenesis* 6(4), 253–64.

Gould, S. J. 1981. *The Mismeasure of Man* New York: W. W. Norton and Co.

Gould, S. J., and R. C. Lewontin. 1978. "The Spandrels of San Marco and the Panglossian Paradigm: A Critique of the Adaptationist Program." *Proceedings of the Royal Society of London* 205, 581–98.

Grady, D. 1997a. 1997b. "Finding Genetic Traces of Jewish Priesthood." *New York Times,* January 7, 1997, sec. C, p. 6, col. 3.

————. 1997b "Brain-Tied Gene Defect May Explain Why Schizophrenics Hear Voices." *New York Times,* January 21, 1997, sec. C, p. 3, col. 1.

Gray, D. S., and G. A. Bray. 1988. "Evaluation of the Obese Patient." In *Handbook of Eating Disorders, Part 2: Obesity,* edited by G. D. Burrows, P. J. V. Beumont, and R. C. Casper. New York: Elsevier.

Greely, H. T. 1992. "Health Insurance, Employment Discrimination, and the Genetics Revolution." In D. J. Kevles and L. Hood, eds., *The Code of Codes: Scientific and Social Issues in the Human Genome Project.* Cambridge, Mass.: Harvard University Press.

Griffiths, P. E., ed. 1992. *Trees of Life.* Boston: Kluwer Academic Publishers.

Griffiths, P. E., and R. D. Gray. 1994. "Developmental Systems and Evolutionary Explanation." *The Journal of Philosophy* 91(6), 277–304.

Griffiths, A. J. F., J. H. Miller, D. T. Suzuki, R. C. Lewontin, and W. M. Gelbart. 1996. *An Introduction to Genetic Analysis.* 6th ed. New York: W. H. Freeman and Co.

Hager, P. 1993. "Justices Cool to O.C. Surrogate Mother's Case." *Los Angeles Times* (Orange County Edition), February 3, 1993, part A, p. 1, col. 5, Metro Desk.

Halaas, J. L., K. S. Gajiwala, M. Margherita, S. L. Cohen, B. T. Chait, D. Rabinowitz, R. L. Lallone, S. K. Burley, and J. M. Friedman. 1995. "Weight-Reducing Effects of the Plasma Protein Encoded by the *Obese* Gene." *Science* 269, 543–46.

Halperin, D. M. 1990. *One Hundred Years of Homosexuality.* New York: Routledge.

Hamer, D. 1995. The Henry R. Luce Professorship of Biotechnology and Society's Symposium: "Genetics and the Human Genome Project: Where Scientific and Public Cultures Meet." Stanford University, November 4, 1995.

Hamer, D., and P. Copeland. 1994. *The Science of Desire.* New York: Simon and Schuster.

————. 1998. *Living with Our Genes: Why They Matter More Than You Think.* New York: Doubleday.

Hamer, D. H., S. Hu, V. L. Magnuson, N. Hu, and A. M. L. Pattatucci. 1993. "A Linkage Between DNA Markers on the X Chromosome and Male Sexual Orientation." *Science* 261, 321–27.

Hazlett, T. W. 1995. "Ding Dong: Intelligence as a Determinant of Achievement." *Reason* 26(8), 66.

Helb, M. R., and T. F. Heatherton. 1998. "The Stigma of Obesity in Women: The Difference Is Black and White." *Personality and Social Psychology Bulletin* 24(4), 417–26.

Henderson, N. D. 1972. "Relative Effects of Early Rearing Environment on Discrimination Learning in Housemice." *Journal of Comparative and Physiological Psychology* 72, 505–11.

Henry, V. L. 1993. "A Tale of Three Women: A Survey of the Rights and Responsibilities of

Unmarried Women Who Conceive by Alternative Insemination and a Model for Legislative Reform." *American Journal of Law and Medicine* 19, 285–305.

Hill, J. L. 1991. "What Does It Mean to Be a 'Parent'? The Claims of Biology as the Basis for Parental Rights." *New York University Law Review* 66, 353–420.

Holden, C. 1987. "The Genetics of Personality." *Science* 237, 598–601.

Hollandsworth, M. J. 1995. "Gay Men Creating Familes Through Surro-Gay Arrangments: A Paradigm for Reproductive Freedom." *American Univeristy Journal of Gender and the Law* 3, 183.

Hood, L. 1992. "Biology and Medicine in the Twenty-First Century." In D. J. Kevles and L. Hood, eds., *The Code of Codes: Scientific and Social Issues in the Human Genome Project.* Cambridge, Mass.: Harvard University Press.

Horgan, J. 1993. "Eugenics Revisited." *Scientific American* 286(6), 122–31.

Horn, J. M., J. C. Loehlin, and L. Willerman. 1979. "Intellectual Resemblance among Adoptive and Biological Relatives: The Texas Adoption Project." *Behavior Genetics* 9(3), 177–201.

Hsia, D. Y. 1970. "Phenylketonuria and Its Variants." In *Progress in Medical Genetics, Volume 7,* edited by A. G. Seinberg and A. G. Bearn. New York: Grune and Stratton.

Hu, S., A. M. Pattatucci, C. Patterson, L. Li, D. W. Fulker, S. S. Cherny, L. Kruglyak, and D. H. Hamer. 1995. "Linkage Between Sexual Orientation and Chromosome Xq28 in Males but Not in Females." *Nature Genetics* 11(3), 248–56.

Hutchinson, G. E. 1965. *The Ecological Theater and the Evolutionary Play.* New Haven: Yale University Press.

Itoh, T., S. Horie, K. Takahanshi, and T. Okubo. 1996. "An Evaluation of Various Indices of Body Weight Change and Their Relationship with Coronary Risk Factors." *International Journal of Obesity Related Metabolic Disorders* 20(12), 1089–96.

———. 1996. "Effects of Weight Cycling on Coronary Risk Factors." *Journal of Epidemiology* 6(1), 55–62.

Jarrett, R. J. 1988. "Epidemiological Studies in Obesity." In *Handbook of Eating Disorders, Part 2: Obesity,* edited by G. D. Burrows, P. J. V. Beumont, and R. C. Casper. New York: Elsevier.

Jeffery, R. W. 1996. "Does Weight Cycling Present a Health Risk?" *American Journal of Clinical Nutrition* 63(3, supplement), 452S–455S.

Jensen, A. R. 1969. "How Much Can We Boost IQ and Scholastic Achievement?" *Harvard Educational Review* 39(15), 1–123.

———. 1980. *Bias in Mental Testing* New York: The Free Press.

———. 1982. "The Limited Plasticity of Human Intelligence" *Eugenics Bulletin* (Fall).

Johnston, T. D., and G. Gottlieb. 1990. "Neophenogenesis: A Developmental Theory of Phenotypic Evolution" *Journal of Theoretical Biology* 147, 471–95.

Judson, H. F. 1992. "A History of the Science and Technology Behind Gene Mapping and Sequencing." In D.J. Kevles and L. Hood, eds., *The Code of Codes: Scientific and Social Issues in the Human Genome Project.* Cambridge, Mass.: Harvard University Press.

Jung, R. T. 1997. "Obesity as a Disease." British Medical Bulletin 53(2), 307–21.

Kagan, J. 1994. *Galen's Prophecy.* New York: Basic Books.

Kassirer, J. P., and M. Angell. 1998. "Losing Weight—An Ill-Fated New Year's Resolution." *The New England Journal of Medicine* 338, 52–54.

Keane, N. P. 1981. *The Surrogate Mother.* New York: Everest House.

Keesey, R. E. 1978. "Set-Points and Body Weight Regulation." In *The Psychiatric Clinics of North America* 1(3), December 1978 *Symposium on Obesity: Basic Mechanisms and Treatment,* edited by A. J. Stunkard, Philadelphia: W. B. Saunders Company.

———. 1988. "The Relation Between Energy Expenditure and the Body Weight Set-Point: Its Significance to Obesity." In *Handbook of Eating Disorders, Part 2: Obesity,* edited by G. D. Burrows, P. J. V. Beumont, and R. C. Casper. New York: Elsevier.

Kendler, K. S. 1998. "Major Depression and the Environment: A Psychiatric Genetic Perspective." *Pharmocopsychiatry* 31, 5–9.

Kendler, K. S. and L. Karkowski-Shuman. 1997. "Stressful Life Events and Genetic Liability to

Major Depression: Genetic Control of Exposure to the Environment?" *Psychological Medicine* 27, 539–47.

Kevles, D. J. 1985. *In the Name of Eugenics: Genetics and the Uses of Human Heredity.* Berkeley and Los Angeles: University of California Press.

Kevles, D. J., and L. Hood, eds. 1992. *The Code of Codes: Scientific and Social Issues in the Human Genome Project.* Cambridge, Mass.: Harvard University Press.

Kitcher, P. 1985, *Vaulting Ambition.* Cambridge, Mass.: MIT Press.

———. 1996. "Behind Closed Doors: Junior Comes Out Perfect," *New York Times,* September 29, 1996 sec. 6, p. 124, col. 1.

———. 2000. "Battling the Undead: How (and How Not) to Resist Genetic Determinism." Forthcoming in R. Singh, C. Drimbas, D. Paul, and J. Beatty, eds., *Thinking about Evolution: Historical, Philosophical, and Political Perspectives.* Cambridge, Mass.: Cambridge University Press.

Klein, R. 1996. *Eat Fat.* New York: Pantheon Books.

Koehler, K. E. 1996. "Artificial Insemination: In the Child's Best Interest?" *Albany Law Journal of Science and Technology* 5, 321.

Kolata, G. 1996. "Is a Gene Making You Read This?" *New York Times,* January 7, 1996, sec. 4, p. 4, col. 1.

———. 1997: "How Fen-Phen, A Diet "Miracle," Rose and Fell." *New York Times,* September 23, 1997, sec. F, p. 1, col. 4.

Koshland, D. E. 1987. "Nature, Nurture, and Behavior." *Science* 235, 1445.

Kramer, P. D. 1993. *Listening to Prozac.* New York: Viking.

Krim, T. M. 1996. "Comparative Health Law: Beyond Baby M: International Perspectives on Gestational Surrogacy and the Demise of the Unitary Biological Mother." *Annuals of Health Law* 5, 193–216.

Laqueur, T. 1990. *Making Sex.* Cambridge, Mass.: Harvard University Press.

Lascarides, D. E. 1997. "A Plea for the Enforceability of Gestational Surrogacy Contracts." *Hofstra Law Review* 25, 1221.

Leary, W. E. 1996. "Scientists Identify Site of Gene Tied to Some Cases of Parkinson's." *New York Times,* November 15, 1996, sec. A, p. 19, col. 1.

Ledley, F. D. 1991. "Clinical Application of Genotypic Diagnosis for Phenylketonuria: Theoretical Considerations." *European Journal of Pediatrics* 150, 752–56.

Le Marchand, L. 1991. "Ethnic Variation in Breast Cancer Survival: A Review." *Breast Cancer Research and Treatment.* May 18, Supplement 1:S, 119–26.

Lesch, K. P., D. Bengel, A. Heils, S. Z. Sabol, B. D. Greenberg, S. Petri, J. Benjamin, C. R. Muller, D. H. Hamer, and D. L. Murphy. 1996. "Association of Anxiety-Related Traits with a Polymorphism in the Serotonin Transporter Gene Regulatory Region." *Science* 274, 1527–31.

Lester, D. 1986. "The Distribution of Sex and Age among Victims of Homicide: A Cross-National Study." *International Journal of Social Psychiatry* 32(2), 47–50.

———. 1991. "Crime as Opportunity." *British Journal of Criminology* 31(2), 186–88.

Levins, R., and R. C. Lewontin. 1985. *The Dialectical Biologist.* Cambridge, Mass.: Harvard University Press.

Lewis-Fernández, R., and A. Kleinman. 1994. "Culture, Personality, and Psychopathology," *Journal of Abnormal Psychology.* 103(1), 67–71.

Lewontin, R. C. 1974. "The Analysis of Variance and the Analysis of Causes," *American Journal of Human Genetics* 26, 400–11. Reprinted in *The Dialectical Biologist* by R. Levins and R. C. Lewontin 1985. Cambridge, Mass.: Harvard University Press.

———. 1978. "Adaptation." *Scientific American,* 239(3).

———. 1982. *Human Diversity* New York: Scientific American Books, Inc.

———. 1993. *Biology as Ideology: The Doctrine of DNA.* HarperPerennial, New York, New York.

Lewontin, R. C., S. Rose, and L. J. Kamin. 1984. *Not in Our Genes.* New York: Pantheon.

Lewontin, R. C., J. A. Moore, W. B. Provine, and B. Wallace, eds. 1981. *Dobzhansky's Genetics of Natural Populations I–XLIII.* New York: Columbia University Press.

Lodgberg, A. 1978. "The Reform of Family Law in the Scandinavian Countries." In A. G. Chloros, ed., *The Reform of Family Law in Europe*. Deventer, Netherlands: Kluwer BV.

Loehlin, J. C. 1992. *Genes and Environment in Personality Development*. Individual Differences and Development Series, vol. 2. Thousand Oaks, Calif.: Sage Publications.

Longino, H. E. 1990. *Science as Social Knowledge*. Princeton, N.J.: Princeton University Press.

Lynch, R. 1993. "Supreme Court Ends O.C. Surrogacy Fight." *Los Angeles Times* (Orange County Edition), October 5, 1993, part A, p. 1, col. 1.

MacDonald, M. 1981. *Mystical Bedlam: Madness, Anxiety, and Healing in Seventeenth-Century England*, Cambridge, Mass.: Cambridge Unversity Press.

Machin, G. A. 1996. "Some Causes of Genotype and Phenotypic Discordance in Monozygotic Twin Pairs." *American Journal of Medical Genetics* 61(3), 216–28.

MacKinnon, C. A. 1984. "Difference and Dominance: On Sex Discrimination." Reprinted in *Feminist Legal Theory*, edited by K. Bartlett and R. Kennedy. 1991. Boulder, Colo.: Westview Press.

Maffei, M., J. Halass, E. Ravussin, R. E. Pratley, G. H. Lee, Y. Zhang, H. Fei, S. Kim, R. Lallone, and S. Ranganathan. 1995. "Leptin Levels in Human and Rodent: Measurement of Plasma Leptin and Ob RNA in Obese and Weight-Reduced Subjects." *Nature Medicine* 1(11). 1155–61.

Malinowski, B. 1916. "Baloma: The Spirits of the Dead in the Trobriand Islands." In Malinowski 1926, 1971, *Myth in Primitive Psychology*. Westpoint, Conn.: Negro University Press.

Mann, C. C. 1994. "Behavioral Genetics in Transition." *Science* 264, 1686–89.

Manson, J. E., W. C. Willett, M. J. Stampfer, G. A. Colditz, D. J. Hunter, S. E. Hankinson, C. H. Hanknekens, and F. E. Speizer. 1995. "Body Weight and Mortality among Women." *New England Journal of Medicine* 333(11), 677–85.

Mark, E. H., and F. R. Ervin. 1970. *Violence and the Brain*. New York, Evanston, and London: Harper and Row.

Marshall, E. 1994. "Manic Depression: Highs and Lows on the Research Roller Coaster." *Science* 264, 1693–95.

Maynard Smith, J. 1981. "Genes and Race." *Nature* 189, 742.

McGuire, M., and A. Troisi. 1998. *Darwinian Psychiatry*. New York: Oxford University Press.

McKinley, J. C., and W. Stevens. 1998. "When Nature Rages: A Special Report." *New York Times*, November 9, 1998, sec. A, p. 1, col. 1.

Moffitt, T. E., and S. A. Mednick. 1988. *Biological Contributions to Crime Causation* (NATO Advanced Study Institute, Series D: Behavioral and Social Sciences—Number 40). Dordrecht, Netherlands: Martinus Nijhoff Publishers.

Moldin, S. O., T. Reich, and J. P. Rice. 1991. "Current Perspectives on the Genetics of Unipolar Depression." *Behavior Genetics* 21(3), 211–42.

Montague, C. T., J. B. Prints, L. Sanders, J. E. Digby, and S. O'Rahilly. 1997. "Depot- and Sex-Specific Differences in Human Leptin mRNA Expression: Implications for the Control of Regional Fat Distribution." *Diabetes* 46, 342–47.

Moore, D. W. 1993. "Public Polarized on Gay Issue." *Gallup Poll Monthly* (April), 30–34.

Morris, C. 1997. "Technology and the Legal Discourse of Fetal Autonomy." *UCLA Women's Law Journal* 8 (Fall/Winter), 47–97.

Muls, E., K. Kempen, G. Vansant, and W. Saris. 1995. "Is Weight Cycling Detrimental to Health? A Review of the Literature in Humans." *International Journal of Obesity Related Metabolic Disorders* 19 (3, supplement), S46–S50.

Murphey, R. M. 1982. "Phenylketonuria (PKU) and the Single Gene: An Old Story Retold." *Behavior Genetics* 13, 141–57.

Murphy, T. F. 1997. *Gay Science: The Ethics of Sexual Orientation Research*. New York: Columbia University Press.

Murray, C. 1997. "IQ Will Put Your in Your Place." *Sunday Times* (UK), May 25, 1997.

Murray, C., and R. J. Herrnstein. 1994. *The Bell Curve*. New York: The Free Press.

Murray, C., and D. Seligman. 1997. "More on the Bell Curve." *National Review*, December 8.

Nelkin, D. 1992. "The Social Power of Genetic Information." In D. J. Kevles and L. Hood, eds., *The Code of Codes: Scientific and Social Issues in the Human Genome Project.* Cambridge, Mass.: Harvard University Press.

Nesse, R. M., and G. C. Williams. 1995. *Why We Get Sick: The New Science of Darwinian Medicine.* New York: Vintage Books.

Nigg, J. T., and H. H. Goldsmith. 1994. "Genetics of Personality Disorders: Perspectives from Personality and Psychopathology Research." *Psychological Bulletin* 115(3), 346–80.

Odling-Smee, F. J. 1988. "Niche-Constructing Phenotypes." In *The Role of Behavior in Evolution,* edited by H. C. Plotkin. Cambridge, Mass.: MIT Press.

Omi, M., and Winant, H. 1986. *Racial Formation in the United States: From the 1960s to the 1980s.* New York: Routledge & Kegan Paul.

———. 1994. *Racial Formation in the United States: From the 1960s to the 1990s.* 2nd ed. New York: Routledge.

Ortiz, O., M. Russell, T. L. Daley, R. N. Baumsartner, M. Waki, S. Lichtman, J. Wang, R. N. Dierson, Jr., and S. B. Heymsfield. 1992. "Differences in Skeletal Muscle and Bone Mineral Mass Between Black and White Females and Their Relevant to Estimates of Body Composition." *American Journal of Clinical Nutrition* 55(1), 8–13.

Oyama, S. 1985. *The Ontogeny of Information.* New York: Cambridge University Press.

Pattatucci, A. M. L., and D. H. Hamer. 1995. "Development and Familiality of Sexual Orientation in Females." *Behavior Genetics* 25(5), 407–20.

Patterson, O. 1995. "For Whom the Bell Curves." Manuscript.

Patzer, G. L. 1985. *The Physical Attractiveness Phenomena.* New York: Plenum Press.

Paul, D. 1994. "Towards a Realistic Assessment of PKU Screening." In D. Hull, M. Forbes, and R. M. Burian, eds., *Proceedings of the Philosophy of Science Association,* vol. 2.

Pelleymounter, M. A., M. J. Cullen, M. B. Baker, R. Hecht, D. Winters, T. Boone, and F. Collins. 1995. "Effects of the *Obese* Gene Product on Body Weight Regulation in *ob/ob* Mice." *Science* 269, 540–43.

Pérusse, L., J. P. Despres, S. Lemieux, T. Rice, D. C. Rao, C. Bouchard. 1996. "Familial Aggregation of Abdominal Visceral Fat Level: results from the Quebec Family Study," *Metabolism* 45(3), 378–82.

Pierce-Gealy, M. 1995. "'Are You My Mother?': Ohio's Crazy-Making Baby-Making Produces a New Definition of "Mother.'" *Akron Law Review* 28 (Spring), 535–60.

Pigliucci, M. 1996. "Modelling Phenotypic Plasticity II: Do Genetic Correlations Matter?" *Heredity* 77, 453–60.

———. 1999. "Ecological and Evolutionary Genetics of *Arabidopsis.*" Forthcoming in *Trends in Plant Science.*

Pigliucci, M., and C. D. Schlichting. 1995. "Reactions Norms of Arabidopsis IV: Relationships Between Plasticity and Fitness." *Heredity* 76, 427–36.

———. 1997. "On the Limits of Quantitative Genetics for the Study of Phenotypic Evolution." *Acta Biotheoretica* 45, 143–60.

Pigliucci, M., and J. Schmitt. 1999. "Genes Affecting Phenotypic Plasticity in *Arabidopsis:* Pleiotropic Effects and Reproductive Fitness of Photomorphogenic Mutants." Forthcoming in *Journal of Evolutionary Biology.*

Pigliucci, M., C. D. Schlichting, C. S. Jones, and K. Schwent. 1996. "Developmental Reaction Norms: The Interactions among Allometry, Ontogeny, and Plasticity." *Plant Species Biology* 11, 69–85.

Pigliucci, M., K. Cammell, and J. Schmitt. 1999a. "Evolution of Phenotypic Plasticity: A Comparative Approach in the Phylogenetic Neighborhood." Forthcoming in *Journal of Evolutionary Biology.*

Pigliucci, M., G. A. Tyler III, and C. D. Schlichtingl. 1999b. "Mutational Effects on Constraints on Character Evolution and Phenotypic Plasticity in *Arabidopsis Thaliana.*" Forthcoming in *Journal of Genetics.*

Platt, S. A., and M. Bach. 1997. "Uses and Misinterpretations of Genetics in Psychology." *Genetica* 99, 135–43.

Plomin, R. 1990. *Nature and Nurture.* Pacific Grove, Calif.: Brooks/Cole Publishing Co.

Plomin, R., J. C. DeFries, and G. E. McClearn. 1990. *Behavioral Genetics: A Primer.* New York: W. H. Freeman and Co.

Plomin, R., J. C. DeFries, G. E. McClearn, and M. Rutter. 1997. *Behavioral Genetics.* 3rd ed. New York: W. H. Freeman and Co.

Plotkin, H. C. 1988. "Behavior and Evolution." In *The Role of Behavior in Evolution,* edited by H. C. Plotkin. Cambridge, Mass.: MIT Press.

Powers, P. S. 1988. "Social Issues in Obesity." In *Handbook of Eating Disorders, Part 2: Obesity* edited by G. D. Burrows, P. J. V. Beumont, and R. C. Casper. New York: Elsevier.

Rasmus, S. J., S. M. Forrest, D. B. Pitt, J. A. Saleeba, and R. G. H. Cotton. 1993. "Comparison of Genotype and Intellectual Phenotype in Untreated PKU Patients." *Medical Genetics* 30, 401–5.

Rice, G., C. Anderson, N. Risch, and G. Ebers. 1999. "Male Homosexuality: Absence of Linkage to Microsatellite Markers at Xq28." *Science* 284, 665–67.

Risch, N., E. Squires-Wheeler, and B. J. B. Keats. 1993. "Male Sexual Orientation and Genetic Evidence." *Science* 262, 2063–65.

Ristow, M., D. Muller-Wieland, A. Pfeiffer, W. Krone, and R. C. Kahn. 1998. "Obesity Associated with a Mutation in Genetic Regulator of Adipocyte Differentiation." *New England Journal of Medine* 339, 953–59.

Satz, D. 1992. "Markets in Women's Reproductive Labor." *Philosophy and Public Affairs* 21(2), (Spring).

Schlichting, C., and M. Pigliucci. 1995. "Gene Regulation, Quantitative Genetics, and the Evolution of Reaction Norms." *Evolutionary Ecology* 8, 1–15.

Schlichting, C. A., and M. Pigliucci. 1998. *Phenotypic Evolution: A Reaction Norm Appro ch.* Sunderland, Mass.: Sinauer Associates, Inc.

Schmitt, J., S. Dudley, and M. Pigliucci. 1999. "Manipulative Approaches to Testing Adaptive Plasticity: Phytochrome-Mediated Shade Avoidance Responses in Plants." Forthcoming in *American Naturalist.*

Schneider, J. 1994. ["Obesity in the Elderly and Very Elderly—Prognostic Significance and Practical Conclusions"]. *Zeitschrift fer Gerontologie* 27(3) (May-June), 208–13.

Scriver, C. 1995. "Whatever Happened to PKU?" *Clinical Biochemistry* 28(2), 137–44.

Scriver, C. R., S. Kaufman, and S. L. C. Woo. 1988. "Mendelian Hyperphenylalaninemia." *Annual Review of Genetics* 22, 301–21.

Selmer, R., and A. Trerdal. 1995. "Body Mass Index and Cardiovascular Mortality at Different Levels of Blood Pressure: A Prospective Study of Norwegian Men and Women." *Journal of Epidemiology and Community Health* 49(3) (June), 256–70.

Shaw, R. 1958. "The Theoretical Genetics of the Sex Ratio." *Genetics* 43, 149–63.

Simopoulos, A. P. 1987. "Characteristics of Obesity: An Overview." In *Annals of the New York Academy of Sciences* 499 (June 15), *Human Obesity,* edited by R. J. Wurtman and J. J. Wurtman. New York: New York Academy of Sciences.

———. 1988. "Characteristics of Obesity." In *Handbook of Eating Disorders, Part 2: Obesity,* edited by G. D. Burrows, P. J. V. Beumont, and R. C. Casper. New York: Elsevier.

———. 1996. "Genetic Variation and Nutrition." *Biomedical and Environmental Sciences* 9, 124–29.

Skyrms, B. 1996. *Evolution of the Social Contract* Cambridge, Mass.: Cambridge University Press.

Sober, E. 1993. *Philosophy of Biology.* San Francisco: Westview Press.

Sober, E., and R. C. Lewontin. 1982. "Artifact, Cause, and Genic Selection." *Philosophy of Science* 49 (June), 157–80.

Steele, C. M. 1997. "A Threat in the Air: How Stereotypes Shape Intellectual Identity and Performance." *American Psychologist* 52(6), 613–29.

———. 1998. "Stereotyping and Its Threat Are Real." *American Psychologist* 53(6), 680–81.

Steele, C. M., and J. Aronson. 1995. "Stereotype Threat and the Intellectual Test Performance of African Americans." *Journal of Personality and Social Psychology* 69(5), 797–811.

Stein, E. 1998. "Essentialism and Constructionism about Sexual Orientation." In *The Philosophy of Biology,* edited by D. L. Hull and M. Ruse. New York: Oxford University Press.

Stevens, J., S. K. Kumanyika, and J. E. Keil. 1994. "Attitudes Toward Body Size and Dieting: Differences Between Elderly Black and White Women." *American Journal of Public Health* 84(8), 1322–25.

Stini, W. A. 1991. "Boby Composition and Longevity: Is There a Longevous Morphotype?" *Medical Anthropology* 13(3) (September), 215–29.

Szasz, T. 1987. *Insanity: The Idea and Its Consequences.* New York: John Wiley and Sons.

Treacy, E., J. J. Pitt, K. Seller, G. N. Thompson, S. Ramus, R. G. H. Cotton. 1996. *"In Vivo* Disposal of Phenylalanine in Phenylketonuria: A Study of Two Siblings." *Journal of Inherited Metabolic Disorders* 19, 595–602.

Tyfield, L. A., A. L. Meredith, M. J. Osborn, R. Primavesi, T. L. Chambers, J. B. Holton, and P. S. Harper. 1990. "Genetic Analysis of Treated and Untreated Phenylketonuria in One Family." *Journal of Medical Genetics* 27, 546–68.

Vigue, L. C. 1996. "Fear of the Inflexible Gene." *American Biology Teacher* 58 (2), 86–88.

Wade, N. 1998. "First Gene to Be Linked with High Intelligence Is Reported Found." *New York Times,* May 14, 1998, sec./ A, p. 16.

Wang, J., J. C. Thorton, M. Russell, S. Burastero, S. Heymsfield, and R. N. Pierson, Jr. 1994. "Asians Have Lower Body Mass Index (BMI) but Higher Percentage Body Fat Than Do Whites: Comparisons of Anthropometric Measurements." *American Journal of Clinical Nutrition* 60(1) (July), 23–28.

Watson, D., and L. A. Clark. 1994. "Introduction to the Special Issue on Personality and Psychopathology." *Journal of Abnormal Psychology* 103(1), 3–5.

Watson, D., L. A. Clark, and A. R. Harkness. 1994. "Structures to Personality and Their Relevance to Psychopathology." *Journal of Abnormal Psychology* 103(1), 18–31.

Watson, J. D. 1992. "A Personal View of the Project." In D. J. Kevles and L. Hood, eds., *The Code of Codes: Scientific and Social Issues in the Human Genome Project.* Cambridge, Mass.: Harvard University Press, 164–76.

———. 1995. Keynote Address, The L. S. B. Leakey Foundation Symposium, "Genetics and Human Evolution," Stanford University, December 2, 1995.

Weiss, W. L. 1997. "Ohio Bill 419: Increased Openness in Adoption Records Law." *Cleveland State Law Review* 45, 101–33.

Wexler, N. 1992. "Clairvoyance and Caution: Repercussions from the Human Genome Project." In D. J. Kevles and L. Hood, eds., *The Code of Codes: Scientific and Social Issues in the Human Genome Project.* Cambridge, Mass.: Harvard University Press, 211–43.

Whitam, F. L., and R. M. Mathy. 1986. *Male Homosexuality in Four Societies.* New York: Praeger Publishers.

Wickelgren, I. 1999. "Discovery of 'Gay Gene' Questioned." *Science* 284, 571.

Widom, C. S. 1991. "A Tail on an Untold Tale: Response to 'Biological and Genetic Contributors to Violence—Widom's Untold Tale.'" *Psychological Bulletin* 109(1), 130–32.

Wilson, E. O. 1975. *Sociobiology: The New Synthesis.* Cambridge, Mass.: Harvard University Press.

———. 1981. "Genes and Racism." *Nature* 289, 627.

Wilson, J. Q., and R. J. Herrnstein. 1985. *Crime and Human Nature.* New York: Simon and Schuster.

Wittgenstein, L. W. c1979. *Remarks on Frazer's Golden Bough,* translated by A. C. Miles, edited by Rush Rhees. Atlantic Highlands, N.J.: Humanities Press International.

Wriggins, J. 1997. "Genetics, IQ, Determinism, and Torts: The Example of Discovery in Lead Exposure Litigation." *Boston University Law Review* 77, 1025–87.

LEGAL CASES CITED

Belsito et al v. Clark et al., 67 Ohio Misc. 2d 54; 644 N.E.2d 760; (1994).

Doe v. Kelley, Mich. App., 307 N.W.2d.

In the Matter of Baby M, 109 N.J. 396; 537 A.2d 1227 (see also N.J. 542 A.2d, 52) (1988).

In Re Marriage of CYNTHIA J. and ROBERT P. MOSCHETTA. CYNTHIA J. MOSCHETTA, Respondent, v. ROBERT P. MOSCHETTA, Appellant; ELVIRA JORDAN, Intervener and Respondent, 25 Cal. App. 4th 1218; 1994 Cal. App. LEXIS 616; 30 Cal. Rptr. 2d 893; 94.

Jhordan C. v. Mary K., 179 Cal. App. 3d386, 224 Cal. Rptr. 530 (1986).

Johnson v. Calvert, 5 Cal. 4th 84; 851 P.2d 776 1993; 19 Cal. Rptr., 2d 494. See also 12 Cal. App. 4th 977 1991; 286 Cal. Rptr. 369. See also *Johnson, I:* Superior Court of Orange County, Nos. X-633190 and AD-57638, Richard N. Parslow, Jr., Judge. See also 510 U.S. 874; 114 S. Ct. 206.

Liston v. Pyles, No. 97APF01-137 1997, Court of Appeals of Ohio, Tenth Appellate District, Franklin County; Lexis 3627.

Matter of Adoption of Baby Girl L.J., N.Y.S., 505 N.Y.S.2d.

Matter of Adoption of Paul, N.Y.S., 550 N.Y.S2d.

McDonald v. McDonald, 196 A.D.2d 7; 608 N.Y.S. 2d 477 (1994).

Surrogate Patenting Associates Inc. v. Commonwealth of Kentucky, ex rel., David Armstrong: Ky., 704 S.W.2d 209.

WORKS WITHOUT BYLINES

"Obesity Genes: Food for Fat Cats" *The Economist*, July 29, 1995, #60.

"Incalculably Inaccurate." *The Economist*, August 20–26, 1994, 332(7877), 22.

"Panic in the Petri Dish." *The Economist*, July 23–29, 1994, 332(7873), 61–62.

"The Future of Medicine." *The Economist*, March 19–25, 1994, 330(7855).

"Boy George, I Think He's Got It." *The Economist*, July 15, 1995, Science and Technology section, 63.

"Double Trouble." *The Economist*, November 18, 1995, Science and Technology section, 89–91.

"Gene May Be Clue to Nature of Nurturing." *New York Times*, July 26, 1996, sec. A, p. 21, col. 1.

INDEX